Treatment of the DSM-III Psychiatric Disorders

William H. Reid, M.D., M.P.H.
Director of Education and Training
Nebraska Psychiatric Institute
University of Nebraska Medical Center
Omaha

With sections by

George U. Balis, M.D.
Institute of Psychiatry and Human Behavior
University of Maryland School of Medicine, Baltimore

and

John Y. Donaldson, M.D.
Nebraska Psychiatric Institite
University of Nebraska Medical Center, Omaha

Brunner/Mazel, *Publishers* • New York

FIFTH PRINTING

Library of Congress Cataloging in Publication Data

Reid, William H., 1945–
    Treatment of the DSM-III psychiatric disorders.

    Includes bibliographies and index.
    1. Mentally ill—Treatment. 2. Psychotherapy.
3. Diagnostic and statistical manual of mental
disorders. 3rd ed. I. Balis, George U.
II. Donaldson, John Y. III. Title. IV. Title:
Treatment of the D.S.M.-III psychiatric disorders.
V. Title: Treatment of the DSM-3 psychiatric disorders.
[DNLM: 1. Mental disorders—Therapy.   WM 400 R359t]
RC480.R4   1983   616.89′1   83-7503
ISBN 0-87630-339-4

Published by
BRUNNER/MAZEL, INC.
19 Union Square West
New York, N.Y. 10003

To Élise, Stephanie and Troy
with love.

Contents

SECTION III *by William H. Reid, M.D., M.P.H.*

Introduction

A great deal of consideration went into the decision to write this book. Questions came to mind about whether there was a need for such a volume, whether and how it might be produced, and whether I was the appropriate author. To the first question the answer is a clear yes. Treatment of psychiatric disorders is an important part of the practice of psychiatric and nonpsychiatric physicians, house officers, and many nonmedical mental health professionals. While this book is intended primarily for physicians, there is a need in all of the clinical fields for a concise volume which focuses solely on treatment guidelines, and which, where appropriate, attempts to integrate the several facets of biological, psychological, family, social, and educational interventions which are useful for our patients. This integration reminds us that these facets of treatment are not additive, but are synergistic.

The question of how to present all of this information has been answered in the format of the pages which follow. The primary author and two other contributors have first assumed that the reader is familiar with psychiatric evaluation and is, in using this book, pursuing treatment approaches with a clear working diagnosis(es) in mind. It is also assumed that the reader has a basic understanding of psychiatry and psychiatric treatment. The text will recommend, describe, and briefly expand upon treatment modalities; however, *we make no effort to present a complete discussion of either general (e.g., "psychotherapy," "neuroleptic medication") or specific (e.g., "systematic desensitization," "haloperidol") treatment modalities.* This book is a guide and not a reference text. Effort has been made to provide up-to-date references; we recommend that the reader consult these and other sources of more detailed information. Finally, treatment modalities which the author considers unproved or experimental are either clearly identified as such or omitted.

An important note: This volume takes the extremely simplistic stance that the disorder to be treated has been accurately diagnosed according to DSM-III criteria. As every clinician knows, initial impressions are not cast in stone. Patient response to a particular treatment may confirm, refute, add to, or have no effect on one's diagnosis. Treatment is dynamic and multifaceted, and not nearly so concrete as might be assumed by a lay reader.

There are certainly more experienced physicians and teachers than this author, who might write a book such as this. Some might prefer that each subsection be written by a different expert, and that the book be an edited volume. I believe that our finished product represents the best compromise of the issues of authorship which might be raised. It is primarily a one-author book; however, major areas of psychiatric treatment for which subspecialty input is absolutely necessary are addressed by experts in those fields, Drs. George U. Balis and John Y. Donaldson.

William H. Reid, M.D., M.P.H.
Nebraska Psychiatric Institute

Acknowledgments

A number of colleagues reviewed sections of the book prior to the final draft. Thanks are due to Drs. James Davis, Stephen Ruedrich, Donald Swanson, and Elizabeth Yager. Medical students Mark James and Lester Lewis assisted in literature searches. As usual, Edna Brooks-Pittman did an outstanding job preparing the manuscript, with assistance from Pam Unruh and Lucille Marshall. Finally, time and facility support from the Nebraska Psychiatric Institute, Merrill T. Eaton, M.D., Director, are gratefully acknowledged.

Treatment of the DSM-III Psychiatric Disorders

Section I

by

John Y. Donaldson, M.D.

Chapter 1

Disorders Usually First Evident in Infancy, Childhood, or Adolescence

MENTAL RETARDATION

Mental retardation is categorized in DSM-III (American Psychiatric Association, 1980) solely by severity of the condition, with each increasing level of DSM-III intellectual impairment representing an additional standard deviation below testing norms. When known, the etiology of the retardation syndrome may suggest various approaches for prevention of treatment (c.f., phenylketonuria, hypothyroidism). In other instances, such as for Down's syndrome, knowing the cause may have little impact on treatment. In these and in idiopathic cases, intervention is based primarily on the psychiatric symptoms compounding the patient's disability.

Retarded children can have any of the psychiatric problems seen in other children, although the most common include Attention Deficit Disorder, Conduct Disorder, and Pervasive Developmental Disorder. Certain psychiatric problems tend to be seen predominantly at a specific level of mental retardation; however, they are by no means exclusively limited to that level.

317.0(x)   Mild Mental Retardation

Persons with this level of retardation are between two and three standard deviations below testing norms (IQ 52–68). The great majority of persons accurately diagnosed as mentally retarded by DSM-III criteria are in this category, and almost all of this group can be managed in the community. Most remain at home during childhood and are usually placed in programs for the educable retarded. They may be placed with normal children in classes such as physical education, music, and art. Persons functioning at lower levels in this group may be placed in programs for the trainable retarded, with less contact with normal peers. They may require some sheltered living or work situation as they become young adults, such as semi-independent living settings or structured, supervised group homes. With proper supervision some of these patients can be competitively employed in unskilled positions. Others will need reduced expectations and increased supervision, such as that found in a sheltered workshop.

The types of psychiatric problems seen most commonly in this group include short attention span, behavior disorders related to poor impulse control, and adjustment disorders associated with anxiety and/or depression. Patients are often subject to ridicule because their relatively normal physical appearance precludes their being easily identified as handicapped by their peers. Treatment of specific emotional disorders in these patients is very similar to treatment of other children with like problems. Medication is occasionally needed to correct Attention Deficit Disorder (see page 8) or Anxiety Disorders (see page 14), but emphasis should be placed on working with families to develop an adequate support system, working with schools to see that the child is appropriately placed and working with the patient directly in a very concrete fashion, to help him or her come to terms with his strengths and limitations, and deal with problems of rejection or ridicule which often occur.

318.0(x)   Moderate Mental Retardation

Patients with Moderate Mental Retardation are between three and four standard deviations below the testing norm (IQ 35–52). They are usually so severely impaired as to be immediately recognizable by the lay public, and may have associated physical deformities or neurologic defects. There is often a disability in language synthesis. Because they are easily recognizable as handicapped, they are somewhat less subject to ridicule than the mildly retarded person, and more often treated with sympathy by siblings and peers. The moderately retarded as a group appear to be more at risk for the development of psychotic conditions or seizure disorders.

When these patients are relatively free of psychiatric complications, they can be maintained at home and in the community if the latter provides sufficient support systems. These may include supervised group homes with high staff-to-patient ratios, behavioral shaping programs, and highly specialized schools and workshops with adequate provision for transportation to them. In most locales patients with this level of disability are eventually institutionalized. The quality of residential programs varies tremendously, and may range from understaffed human warehouses to truly enlightened programs which provide meaningful activities, supervision, and asylum (in the classical sense of that word) from the pressures of the outside world.

The most common reason for the institutionalization of the moderately retarded patient is his or her tendency to develop a serious psychiatric illness, such as schizophrenia associated with severe temper outbursts. These patients often have idiosyncratic reactions to medication, because of their organic CNS dysfunction. They are particularly prone to paradoxical response such as disinhibition of temper associated with phenothiazines. Haloperidol is often effective for the treatment of emotional dyscontrol in this group. The dosage may be as little as 0.5 mg per day, but can be considerably higher. With good response to neuroleptic medication and adequate community support, many more of these patients are able to remain in the community than was the case 15 or 20 years ago.

Many moderately retarded patients respond quite well to behavior modification programs, either in group homes or in an institutional setting. These may be at least as effective as medication in controlling inappropriate behaviors, especially when the behaviors are annoying but not dangerous, or when they are due to physiologic dysfunction. The best programs frequently contain immediate, concrete rewards which can be clearly associated with the desired behavior.

318.1(x)   Severe Mental Retardation

These patients represent the group between four and five standard deviations below testing norms (IQ 20–35). They are rarely seen in the ordinary psychiatric practice.

Severely retarded patients typically have almost total impairment of language and many associated physical stigmata, although most are ambulatory. They are usually not maintained in the community except as preadolescent children. They may suffer marked delay in physical development. Some will require psychiatric intervention as early as age three or four because of sleep disturbances, temper outbursts, or severe hyperactivity which may be associated with autistic-like behaviors. These usually respond to neuroleptic medications, but the clinician should be alert to the great variability in dosage needs and individual response to specific medication.

In addition to utilizing psychotropic medication when indicated, one must help the patient's parents to work with available support systems such as special education programs. The family must make plans for the child's long-term care and so should receive the best possible information with respect to ability of services for children at this level of impairment.

318.2(x)   Profound Mental Retardation

These patients have IQs below 20, five or more standard deviations below testing norms. They are a small group and are almost all in specialized care programs from an early age because of physical and intellectual impairment. Many have a shortened life span. They rarely cause enough disturbance, because of their inability to move or be active, to attract the attention of a psychiatrist. They are much more likely to need help with intractable seizures or other severely debilitating medical problems. Most treatment programs involve the total care of children who need help with feeding and toileting and are unable to engage in any meaningful activity or interaction.

319.0(x)   Unspecified Mental Retardation

This category is used most often for very young or severely psychotic children who appear to be retarded but are impossible to accurately evaluate. These children are usually ultimately found to be moderately or severely retarded. Treatment of the frequently present childhood psychosis (see page 30) will often help make the child more easily testable and may in some cases improve functional intellectual capacity.

In all groups of retarded children one of the most important services of the psychiatrist is to facilitate the resolution of the parents' grief. In situations in which grief has not occurred, there is a great tendency for some parents to deny the severity of the child's impairment, and with this to waste a great deal of time in efforts to find cures or to vent anger at various helping organizations who are limited in their ability to repair the damage.

ATTENTION DEFICIT DISORDER

314.01   Attention Deficit Disorder with Hyperactivity

Attention Deficit Disorder with Hyperactivity is approximately equivalent to syndromes described by older terms such as "hyperkinetic reaction of childhood" or "minimal cerebral dysfunction." Most children with this diagnosis combine relatively low levels of physiologic arousal with a degree of very slight and typically diffuse, nonspecific neurologic impairment. In addition to determining whether the child meets DSM-III diagnostic criteria, it is extremely important to assess his or her physiologic state. Most of these children will respond to stimulant or antidepressant medication. A few will be made worse by these medications and will improve on tranquilizers. Physiologic assessment helps predict which type of intervention is most likely to be helpful and prevent undesirable reactions to medication.

In addition to the DSM-III criteria for Attention Deficit Disorder, a child likely to respond to stimulant medication will be relatively free of physiologic signs of anxiety. He will tend to have warm, dry hands even under stress, relatively hypoactive reflexes, little if any history of functional gastrointestinal or genitourinary symptoms, and will often be an early riser. These children often seem to crave excitement.

They may temporarily look much better when they are under stress, such as when confronted or in a one-to-one tutorial setting, but will show disinhibition of their behavior when left to themselves. Some studies have shown them to have lower than average levels of biogenic amines and other key neurotransmitters. Stimulant or antidepressant medication seems to increase the child's capacity to inhibit him- or herself, improve overall attention span and ability to maintain internal thought processes in spite of external distraction, and decrease some of their need for excitement or thrill-seeking behavior.

A child of this type at a preschool age will often respond positively to 5 mg of methylphenidate given with breakfast and lunch, or to 5 mg of dextroamphetamine in "spansule" form. By about age seven most of these children need 15–20 mg of methylphenidate (or 10 mg of dextroamphetamine) per day in divided doses. Methylphenidate is now available in 20 mg sustained release form for once-a-day dosage. Occasionally, it is necessary to use higher drug levels; however, many authorities feel that there is usually little to be gained and unacceptable risk of adverse effects. The clinician must be alert for any side effects and tolerance. Some children will develop insomnia, many will show poor appetite, and some will have problems with impaired growth. This is of special concern when the patient is expected to be on medication for several years. Dextroamphetamine appears to have a more serious tendency to slow growth than does methylphenidate. Methylphenidate is commonly chosen over dextroamphetamine in part because of its more acceptable range of side effects and in part because it seems to augment the actions of dopamine and norepinephrine. Because of this effect it may be more likely to be helpful with learning defects of a visual-perceptual nature. Dextroamphetamine is often more useful when hyperactivity or deficit in attention is a more serious problem than learning disability.

Occasionally, pemoline may be used as an alternative medication. However, several studies have indicated that it is slightly less effective than methylphenidate and is, in most children, at least as likely to cause side effects. Some children respond well to the antidepressant medication, imipramine. Often a child who also has had a bed-wetting problem will show a positive behavioral response when placed on imipramine. Usually the patient can be continued on a low dose for several years without significant effects on appetite or growth. Many children under the age of seven will respond to 10 mg per day of imipramine. Most children over seven will require 25 mg. Occasionally, patients approaching adolescence will no longer respond positively to stimulant medication; often imipramine will prove to be more effective for that age group.

A few children who meet DSM-III standards for Attention Deficit Disorder with Hyperactivity will have intense physiologic signs of anxiety. In addition to having cold, sweaty hands, hyperactive reflexes, frequent histories of functional stomachaches, etc., these children often have a history of great difficulty initiating sleep and a tendency to play well by themselves but to become fidgety and hyperexcitable in a group setting. Most tend to do poorly with one-to-one tutorial efforts to correct school problems. They seem to have poor stress tolerance. A child of this type who is placed on stimulant medication will usually become withdrawn. This may be initially mistaken for improvement, but in time it becomes apparent that the child continues to have poor appetite, disturbed sleep, and often a tendency to become explosively aggressive. The aggression is different from the thrill-seeking behavior sometimes seen in the low anxiety group described earlier. It often has an almost paranoid quality and may be a major cause of a shift of care from pediatrician to child psychiatrist.

Children who have this anxious physiology will frequently respond well to efforts to reduce their anxiety. Sometimes this can be done through restructuring of the child's environment or through individual or family psychotherapy. Occasionally it is necessary to use some type of neuroleptic medication, especially when the patient begins to exhibit the type of aggressive behavior described above.

Minor tranquilizers such as the benzodiazepines are not recommended for chronically anxious children unless used very briefly to deal with situational stress. If it is essential to use medication on a long-term basis, these children will often respond positively to very low doses of high-potency neuroleptic medication (such as ½–1 mg of haloperidol per day or 1 mg of fluphenazine). If associated aggression is severe, sedative phenothiazines in the range of 25–100 mg per day (chlorpromazine equivalent), in divided doses, may be used. Extrapyramidal side effects are not usually a problem at these levels, but one should be especially alert to the development of akathisia or other subtle forms.

A few children seem to combine intense physiologic levels of anxiety with minimal brain dysfunction. These patients seem to be especially predisposed toward poor response to medication, or perhaps a very narrow therapeutic window. It is not uncommon to see a child of this type become extremely anxious and possibly overtly disorganized when given stimulant medication, and then disinhibited with more severe impairment of attention when placed on any type of major tranquilizer. Very careful titration of dosage may be useful. A few children afflicted in this way will do better on a combination of medications; some become worse with any drug. Others seem to improve with the elimination of certain foods, food colors, or preservatives from their diet. Many of these patients will also require a variety of social interventions such as described below.

Many of these patients will require careful structuring of their time and environment so as to minimize the adverse consequences of impulsive behavior, rash decision-making, and the like. Children with Attention Deficit Disorder often require the careful listing of rules. They seem to need frequent reminders of their goals and the purpose for pursuing a particular activity. These patients are especially at risk of becoming alienated from parents, teachers, and other adult authority figures. Care can be taken to prevent as much of this as possible, but for the more severely afflicted it seems to be an almost inevitable consequence of the disorder. Many patients will achieve at lower educational and socioeconomic levels than their parents or siblings in spite of efforts to treat their disorder. One should therefore think more in terms of working to minimize disability and helping the child maintain positive relationships with key figures in his or her life. Although there is some tendency for symptoms of hyperactivity to be outgrown with adolescence, inattention and impulsivity frequently remain and may require special support and guidance throughout adolescence and the young adult years.

314.00   Attention Deficit Disorder without Hyperactivity

This is considered by many authorities to be essentially the same disorder as Attention Deficit Disorder with Hyperactivity. Certainly, severe attention problems are present in children who are not hyperactive. This pattern is more likely to be seen in young girls, whose incessant talking causes problems in school. The majority of the patients will respond favorably to stimulants or antidepressant medication as noted in the section above. With any child who manifests an Attention Deficit Disorder without Hyperactivity, one should be alert to associated problems with high levels of anxiety (as noted above) or to the possibility of an incipient schizophrenic process. Either might be more appropriately treated with low doses of neuroleptics.

314.80   Attention Deficit Disorder, Residual Type

This disorder is more likely to be seen in adolescents and young adults who manifested inattention, impulsivity, and hyperactivity as children and who continued to show some symptoms after puberty. A few of these patients will require stimulant medication, although the risk of abuse and sale to other peers becomes greater in adolescence and young adulthood. More will respond positively to antidepressants, especially if there is associated antisocial behavior.

CONDUCT DISORDER

312.00   Conduct Disorder, Undersocialized, Aggressive

This is the most severe of the conduct disorders, the most commonly diagnosed, and tends to have the poorest prognosis. All persons who are eventually diagnosed as having Antisocial Personality Disorder as adults met the criteria for this diagnostic category either in childhood or adolescence, although not all Conduct Disorder patients grow up to be antisocial.

Individual and family psychotherapy appear to be of limited benefit; in most patients the greatest emphasis should be placed on physiologic and social interventions. Family therapy may be appropriate in cases in which the child remains in an intact and competent family setting. Typically, such treatment primarily involves efforts to support the parents and help them learn not to be divided by the actions of the child. The professional may help them develop contingency plans for different levels of misbehavior. Highly motivated parents can provide enough structure to successfully maintain many of these patients within the home environment until they complete or drop out of school; however, many will eventually require some type of outside intervention.

A few patients will respond to pharmacologic interventions which attempt to increase their often very low anxiety to more normal levels. This may decrease the need for thrill-seeking behavior and increase tolerance of ordinary activities, as well as the patient's capacity to learn from experience. The most commonly used medication is imipramine. This tricyclic antidepressant can be effective in very low doses in children and adolescents, often in the range of 10–50 mg per day. A disproportionate number of children with Conduct Disorder are also enuretic; for reasons not fully understood, the best clinical response to imipramine seems to occur in patients who have had a history of, but not necessarily concomitant, bed-wetting.

Imipramine doses of 75 mg per day or more in adolescent patients should be used with considerable caution. Some studies have indicated a tendency toward elevated blood pressure and cardiac rhythm disturbances when higher levels are used in patients this age. Ideally the medication should be titrated to create mild physiologic signs of anxiety but not undue fearfulness. Since these patients have a poor tolerance for very high levels of anxiety, they may be at increased risk for explosive aggression should anxiety become excessive.

It should be noted that a small number of patients who meet the behavioral criteria for Conduct Disorder have unusually high levels of anxiety. This subgroup may fight out of fear and may react with explosive violence when under stress. Some of these anxious aggressive patients will respond positively to low doses of high-potency neuroleptic medications such as halo-peridol, chlorpromazine, or thiothixene. Titration of dosage is important, as excessive medication may cause some patients to become disinhibited and appear much as the non-anxious subgroup of undersocialized aggressive patients. It should be stressed that the majority of patients with this diagnosis are not significantly improved by medication and other means of treatment must be found.

It is frequently necessary to work with the juvenile court to place the patient in some type of structured environment. The number and quality of alternative placement programs vary tremendously from community to community. Some simply provide a higher level of supervision than is found in a chaotic home. Others provide considerable evening and weekend structure but allow public school attendance. The most highly structured provide a 24-hour program including specialized schooling. The latter is often only one step away from some form of incarceration such as a training school or youth development center.

Group homes or structured environments are frequently stressful. This seems to be helpful for the majority of Conduct Disorder patients who have abnormally low levels of anxiety, but occasionally one may see increased violent behavior in the high anxiety subgroup. A limited number of patients improve after a period of care in such an environment. For many others the experience has only provided a protective setting.

Although many mental health professionals are ambivalent about placing a patient in such a structured environment, especially considering the limited potential for significant improvement and the possibility that some patients may actually become worse, this author feels that one should not hesitate to use highly structured settings when necessary. Such a program might, for example, be considered when a severely undersocialized, aggressive patient is not improving on an adolescent inpatient psychiatric unit, threatens to be destructive to the program or other patients, and continues to be too defiant to return home. Such decisions should not be made lightly; however, if serious problems remain after several weeks in the treatment setting, placement elsewhere may be more useful.

312.10   Conduct Disorder, Undersocialized, Nonaggressive
Patients with this diagnosis are relatively rare in psychiatric practice, and may represent a milder form of the undersocialized, aggressive type of Conduct Disorder. In spite of their lack of violent behavior, these children and

adolescents are often seen in juvenile court because of their frequent involvement in nonaggressive violations or "status" offenses. Antidepressant medication may be tried, using the guidelines in the previous section. These patients can often be maintained in the home if extra effort is made to provide adequate supervision. When it is necessary to place them in a group setting, they usually do fairly well.

312.23   Conduct Disorder, Socialized, Aggressive
This disorder is probably the most rarely seen in psychiatric practice of the four major subgroups of Conduct Disorder. Its definition implies a normal capacity for interpersonal attachment but a significant loyalty to a peer group for which the behavioral norm is aggression and delinquency. The capacity for attachment and tolerance of structure allow better response to psychotherapeutic intervention and/or residential placement. Social interventions such as special school programs and family therapy aimed at increasing structured guidance are appropriate treatment approaches.

312.21   Conduct Disorder, Socialized, Nonaggressive
As is the case with several of the other conduct disorders, children in this diagnostic category are more likely to come to the attention of juvenile authorities than psychiatrists. These patients are more often from intact, or at least adequate, families. Outpatient treatment and work with the family, aimed at providing greater supervision and filling the patient's time with appropriate activities, may be useful.

312.90   Atypical Conduct Disorder
Patients with Conduct Disorder who do not fulfil criteria for one of the four major subtypes should be treated based upon presenting symptoms, family and social setting, and underlying psychodynamics, using the principles outlined in earlier sections.

ANXIETY DISORDERS OF CHILDHOOD OR ADOLESCENCE

309.21   Separation Anxiety Disorder
Parents of children with Separation Anxiety Disorder are not likely to seek help for their affected child until sometime during latency. Separation difficulty may be manifested in the early grades, but the presentation of this disorder seems to be most frequent just prior to adolescence. Severity varies considerably from the relatively minor case which responds to gentle encouragement

to extreme conditions that prevent months of school attendance and require almost constant presence of the parents.

Treatment depends to a large extent on the clinician's concept of the disorder's underlying etiology. The majority of patients come from one or more of three categories: psychogenic, constitutional (often with anxious temperament), and depressive.

In families in which the psychogenic causes are most significant, there is often an older, lonely, perhaps depressed parent who was ambivalent about having the child. Mixed messages lead to the child's uncertainty about his or her status within the family. Like the unsure employee who never goes on vacation for fear of being replaced, these children seem to cling desperately to their position in the family. In other cases, the parent may see the world as a hostile and forbidding place, and communicate that fear to the child. Often such a parent is more than willing to have the child remain at home and provide company.

Treatment of such cases should include individual psychotherapy and family therapy as part of an effort to improve the child's self-esteem and relationships and communication within the family. The child should be made to feel more secure, and should be desensitized to the prospect of separation. Although a hospital setting is sometimes required, treatment can take place at home if the parent shows good ego strength and problems are mild to moderate. The child typically shows signs of panic at the time of separation which rapidly subside once the break has occurred. Although it may recur with each separation (such as when going to school), if the parent persists the child will usually develop increasing confidence in his or her ability to deal with separation.

A small percentage of children with Separation Anxiety Disorder are innately anxious and appear to become aversively conditioned by almost any "bad thing" that happens to them at school, in the neighborhood, on the playground, etc. Although separation difficulty appears to be the problem, genuine fears about the dangers of the real world are more at issue. Some such patients may respond to psychotherapy or other techniques aimed at reducing their overall level of anxiety; however, many have such high levels of anxiety that medication may be necessary. Those patients who need drugs typically have almost constant physiologic signs of anxiety such as cold sweaty hands, hyperreflexia, and psychophysiologic discomfort.

Low doses of benzodiazepines may be used temporarily; chronic use should be avoided. Children who have chronic severe problems, with associated symptoms of extreme obsessiveness or suggestion of thought disorder, may respond to low doses of neuroleptic medication (e.g., trifluoperazine, 1–

2 mg per day) as part of an effort to lower their susceptibility to aversive stimuli. These patients need the same level of support, psychotherapy, and encouragement as do those with more prominently psychogenic problems. It should be stressed that antianxiety drugs should not be used to treat the acute panic associated with separation. The main purpose of the medication is to decrease background anxiety sufficiently to allow the child to enjoy exploring new activities on his or her own.

A somewhat larger group of patients appear to have Separation Anxiety which is a symptom of depression. In contrast to the extremely anxious child, the patient who has a "depressive equivalent" is usually free of physiologic signs of anxiety except during times when separation is imminent. Low-to-moderate doses of tricyclic antidepressants may be useful. Effective doses are generally at or below 75 mg of imipramine. Reports of patients whose doses were increased to high levels (e.g., 450 mg of amitriptyline) indicate little therapeutic usefulness and significant, occasionally lethal, cardiac side effects. Any child treated with antidepressant medication should be carefully monitored for physiologic signs of anxiety, sleep disturbance, and other adverse effects.

313.21   Avoidant Disorder of Childhood or Adolescence

These extremely shy children appear to suffer from a continuation and exaggeration of the "stranger anxiety" which is normal in toddlers. This eventually interferes not only with the child's relationships with adults, but also with interaction among peers. It is not uncommon to find that an older sibling or parent has been quite critical of the patient, and has caused some impairment in self-confidence and willingness to reach out toward others. Many milder forms of the disorder are tolerated by families and schools and are not treated. More severe cases may become disabling and impede development, particularly in latency.

The main goal of treatment should be to identify the source of the child's anxiety and to relieve it. Many children will respond to a mixture of individual and family psychotherapy. The absence of global anxiety suggests that the disorder is not related to a constitutional predisposition, and decreases the likelihood that medication will be helpful.

One should be alert to the possibility of a more pervasive disorder, including latent thought disorder. A subgroup of patients with Avoidant Disorder may be at risk for much more serious psychopathology as they mature. If indications of serious developmental delay related to the extreme aloneness are seen, the careful use of psychotropic medications may be indicated. The more potent neuroleptics may be used in doses of approximately 1–2 mg per day, combined with appropriate psychotherapy and family intervention.

313.00   Overanxious Disorder

Patients with this disorder appear clinically to be overly apprehensive, to tolerate stress poorly, and often to have difficulty initiating sleep because of obsessive replaying of the events of the day or some other worry. When the level of anxiety is not disabling, it may be associated with better-than-average intellectual ability, sensitivity, and creativity. These children are seldom aggressive in a thrill-seeking sense, but may strike out when they feel cornered or under pressure.

Several different treatment modalities may be helpful. The child may have been raised in a relatively controlled environment and taught to inhibit motor activity and other means of discharging tension. He or she may respond to efforts to increase assertiveness and overall activity level. Other patients have significant emotional conflicts which require psychotherapeutic intervention, either individually or with emphasis on the family. Psychotherapy should be aimed at helping the child to understand his or her underlying feelings and the conflicts that are present about their expression.

For many patients the high level of anxiety appears to represent a constitutional predisposition toward anxious temperament. Most of these children can be managed without medication; however, those who have disabling levels of anxiety, who become severely aggressive, or who experience serious problems with concentration or obsessive behavior may require pharmacologic intervention. The most severe of these states may be near-psychotic; these patients may respond to very low doses of high potency neuroleptic medication. Positive response should be associated with increased sociability, more openness, and a gradual ability to become more normally assertive. Withdrawal of the medication may be possible once more appropriate habits and behavior patterns have become established.

Some children continue to require medication for several years. The dosage requirement may increase with puberty. Judicious use of neuroleptic drugs may prevent serious decompensation in the small percentage of patients who are predisposed to more serious psychiatric illness as they enter the teen years; however, it should be stressed that such an approach should be reserved for the most severely affected children.

OTHER DISORDERS OF INFANCY, CHILDHOOD, OR ADOLESCENCE

313.89   Reactive Attachment Disorder of Infancy

This category is approximately synonymous with failure to thrive or hospitalism. It correlates with a lack of adequate maternal care and stimulation more than with any defect in the child. Clearly, then, the appropriate intervention in this type of situation is to identify the cause of the maternal deprivation and attempt to correct it. This may prove to be depression or psychosis in the primary caretaker, or a simple lack of parenting skills and a need for training and supervision of a very young or an intellectually impaired mother. It may also be due to more serious problems in the parent, who may be poorly motivated for change.

In extreme cases a substitute caretaker must be provided. This may be suggested by a hospital evaluation in which no physical cause for the child's poor development is found, and during which marked improvement in the child's functional abilities is noted. It is usually necessary to involve a social agency, or possibly the courts, to help provide an adequate alternative caretaker.

These patients are usually treated by pediatricians. A psychiatrist may be asked to see the child as part of a hospital consultation.

313.22   Schizoid Disorder of Childhood or Adolescence

Schizoid Disorder of Childhood or Adolescence is, in effect, a more severe and pervasive form of the Avoidant Disorder (313.21). These patients may have confused thinking and are not only shy, but also very outspoken about their desire to have minimal contact with others while pursuing frequently idiosyncratic interests. There is a high risk for serious social impairment and emotional illness as they mature. Not all develop schizophrenia, but nearly all patients with "process" schizophrenia have had this type of early life history.

Therapy should focus largely on attempting to build a bridge of attachment with these children. Individual and family therapy will often make it possible to discover likely causes of the child's withdrawal and also give some indication of his or her potential for relationships with others. If psychogenic factors appear to be primary, individual and/or family therapy should be continued according to the dynamics of the case.

Some patients, especially those from intact, fairly healthy families, may have subtle neurologic impairment. In these situations, the clinician should carefully assess the child for "soft" neurologic signs, thoroughly explore the early developmental history for indications of cerebral insult or infection, and consider obtaining neuropsychological assessment. If such studies suggest a structural organic basis for the child's difficulty, one might emphasize either medical intervention or some type of specialized behavioral program to meet the child's educational needs and identify areas of potential success.

Finally, it would appear that some patients are strongly physiologically predisposed toward poor stress tolerance and have withdrawn from human interaction as a means of coping with the unpleasant feelings they associate with such interactions. A subgroup of these patients may respond to low doses of high-potency neuroleptic medication such as haloperidol, trifluoper-azine, fluphenazine or thiothixene. Early treatment in this manner has some potential to minimize associated developmental abnormalities, although the child may remain at physiologic risk to decompensate under stress during adolescence or young adulthood. The risk may be less if, because of treatment, there has been an opportunity to develop some significant relationships and normal peer group activities during critical stages of latency and adolescence.

313.23   Elective Mutism

Although rare, Elective Mutism stands out in the minds of many clinicians because the children appear so normal but are usually so difficult to treat. Since the patient typically will not speak to anyone except a few family mem-bers, family and other sources of collateral information are extremely impor-tant. Often there has been a time of considerable dependence on a parent or older sibling who has spoken for the child. In some patients this has been compounded by a traumatic public incident in which the child was placed in a power struggle with an adult who insisted that he or she speak. One may ex-plain to the child one's hypothesis about the nature of his or her disorder and its origins, and talk about the need to speak to other people so that his or her needs can be communicated. If time, distance, and financial factors are not limiting, it may be possible for the psychiatrist to undertake the lengthy pro-cess of desensitization toward speech. It is often sufficient to confirm the di-agnosis and develop an overall treatment plan which can be carried out by others (a speech therapist, school counselor, special education teacher, etc.). Patients may be taught to give short responses in individual sessions, then gradually to widen their sphere of self-expression, for example with the thera-pist and a parent, therapist and a best friend, and eventually a larger number of friends.

As in other children with phobic-like anxiety disorders, one may see a broad range of contributing etiologic factors. In some cases psychogenic fac-tors may be relatively more significant and be best treated with some combi-nation of family and individual therapy, in addition to the efforts focused primarily on the speech disturbance. In others, the patients may be so obvi-ously anxious that medication may be in order. In still others, an associated Separation Anxiety Disorder may respond to the low doses of antidepressant medication described in that section.

313.81   Oppositional Disorder

Like obsessive-compulsive adults, these patients tend to be extremely rigid and defensive about their behavior. Usually the defiance is not overt in the sense that the patients step totally outside of the expected norm. Instead, they behave as though compelled to justify their position—to prove the correctness of their position and the incorrectness of that of an authority figure.

Psychotherapy should focus primarily on discovering underlying sources of anger. Often the therapist becomes a focal point for the child's anger as he or she perceives the therapist as his or her ultimate authority figure. Rogerian or Adlerian approaches seem particularly helpful. Paradoxical intent may occasionally be used; however, caution is recommended. The ability of the therapist to inject humor into the situation can be effective in breaking the ice with these patients. They have commonly had a very serious parent who has provided a model for compulsive behavior and the need to justify every position taken.

In family therapy, emphasis should be placed on helping the parent to modify his or her approach to the child. Patients and their parents tend to be very sensitive to who is "winning" and who is "losing." One should avoid situations in which either the parent or the child is placed in a position of "losing face." In time, both sides will learn to give ground gracefully, but this can only be done after the child and the parent have developed a close and trusting relationship with the therapist.

313.82   Identity Disorder

Late adolescent patients with Identity Disorder have a severe and more intense crisis about the key issues of identity that are normally resolved during the early teen years and/or in the final stages of formal education. Psychotherapy, sometimes relatively intensive and long-term, is frequently helpful. Its emphasis should be on helping these patients to discover deep interests and sources of pleasure. Since many patients make extensive use of splitting, part of psychotherapy should help them learn to deal with the ambivalence that is inherent in becoming more accepting of life's imperfections and compromises. Reducing high levels of anxiety may help patients to cope with ambivalence with a decreased sense of urgency. The anxiety may be relieved by physical activity, psychotherapy, or by judicious use of anxiety-relieving medications. In cases where paralyzing levels of ambivalence exist in association with high levels of anxiety, low doses of neuroleptics may be helpful.

A group of patients may have inertia due to endogenous depression. Adolescents respond to relatively low doses of antidepressants; often 25–75 mg of imipramine or its equivalent will increase activity levels significantly. Antidepressants are usually not helpful in patients who have intense physiologic signs of anxiety. With this group, one should be alert to the possibility of a schizophrenic process which could be made worse by the use of antidepressant medication.

EATING DISORDERS

307.10 Anorexia Nervosa

Although hospitalization is unnecessary for many patients with Anorexia Nervosa, it is prudent to review the inpatient management of severe manifestations of this sometimes life-threatening disorder. Hospitalization may have a number of goals, including providing support and dietary control, instituting a medication regimen, and emergency treatment when the patient has become so emaciated that hyperalimentation or other measures are necessary. The latter should be done in consultation with a physician experienced in internal medicine.

Although sometimes necessary, hospitalization and related treatment methods have a disadvantage of drawing the clinician into a power struggle with the patient.

During the acute inpatient phase of treatment, behavior modification techniques are often the most appropriate treatment approach. These should be applied within a rigidly consistent setting, preferably one in which the staff is experienced in the treatment of anorexic patients. Reinforcers and goals are carefully established. Such programs tend to be highly successful in restoring weight; however, it must be realized that they are not likely to be curative in the sense that the patient will retain normal eating patterns.

It is often productive to teach patients about nutrition and a balanced approach to eating; however, the staff must avoid being drawn into lengthy discussions of food by the patient, who is attempting to avoid underlying issues of aloneness, battles for control, lack of direction, and the like.

Medical interventions are important in several ways. The fasting process itself may create some abnormality in physiology that perpetuates the disorder. Some patients appear to have a combination of high anxiety, marked peripheral vasospasm, and almost no appetite which responds to noradrenergic blocking medication such as chlorpromazine. Another subgroup, with what seems to be early satiety rather than true lack of appetite, may respond to low doses of a dopamine blocker, which seems to improve the distorted body image and decrease excessive rumination about food.

Some other patients may have depression sufficient to necessitate antidepressant medication. Patients who are less obsessive in speech and thinking style appear most likely to respond to this class of drugs.

Medication should be seen either as helping to correct a physiologic imbalance associated with the starvation process, or as an aid in correcting some long-standing source of discomfort. The use of medication should always be combined with individual and family therapy aimed at dealing with basic psychologic issues of fear and control, distortion of body image, strengthening the structure of the family (when the patient lives at home), and discussing transference feelings (which often appear around the issue of medication) and the decision to continue with treatment. The latter is mentioned because deep emotional issues are the most significant cause of anorexic patterns in these patients, and insight-oriented psychotherapy is the most useful treatment modality for many patients.

It should be stressed that many patients with Anorexia Nervosa have features of the borderline personality (q.v.). The therapeutic relationship is likely to be long and stormy; however, continued success may depend upon the presence of a single, consistently available therapist.

307.51   Bulimia

Although listed separately from Anorexia Nervosa in DSM-III, Bulimia is often combined with it in some way. Vomiting associated with Bulimia may in time cause enough weight loss to meet the criteria for Anorexia Nervosa and it is not unusual for patients formerly suffering from anorexia to adopt bulimic eating patterns as a means of meeting both their food cravings and their need to maintain a certain, often unrealistically low, ideal weight. There is considerable similarity in the psychodynamics of both disorders.

Intervention may be approached at several levels. Many patients are depressed and will respond to antidepressant medication. Some have poor eating habits and find that they are able to prevent their intense craving if they follow a diet plan that includes a pattern of more frequent, small meals. For some a gain in weight to a level more typical for their height, but short of excessive weight, will reduce the cravings. Groups such as Overeaters Anonymous provide support which is helpful to some patients. Eating disorder clinics, now available in many cities, utilize support and behavioral programs. One of these may be the best early choice for treatment, provided the staff is professional and experienced.

For the many patients who have already tried several lay approaches to stop their binges, consistent and accepting psychotherapy is recommended. This should provide a solid transference upon which issues of loss, filling emotional voids, having control over gratifying objects, and expression of strong feelings all come to be seen as represented in the bulimic behavior. In such treatment the binges must be seen as having a defensive purpose, such as repression of anger. Recurrences must be tolerated by the therapist and not continuously focused upon, while exploration of other social and emotional material takes place.

Occasionally, patients develop such intense vomiting that serious electrolyte disturbances occur. This may also occur with associated laxative abuse. The most common is depletion of potassium. Patients vomiting several times a day should be closely monitored for this and other complications which are indications for hospitalization. In an inpatient setting the patient can be observed after eating, allowing the majority of food to pass the pylorus before the patient has an opportunity to induce vomiting. After the patient has had several satisfactory meals and reestablished normal electrolyte balance, there is often a decrease in the drive to binge. At this point greater focus can be placed on individual and family psychotherapy, and medication.

It is not uncommon for patients to have bulimic episodes after alcohol abuse. It is therefore important for the clinician to consider helping the patient learn to drink appropriately or abstain as a means of helping to control his or her bulimic impulses.

307.52   Pica

This is a relatively rare disorder which should not be diagnosed if it is associated with another emotional disturbance such as autism or Klein-Levin syndrome. It is usually seen in children of preschool age and lower socioeconomic background. There appears to be some association between this disorder and poor supervision and/or certain mineral deficiencies. Patients should be evaluated for trace mineral deficiency, especially iron and zinc, and should also be assessed for abnormally high levels of lead. Any deficiencies found should be corrected. In some patients this alone will alleviate the problem. In others the major focus of treatment should involve efforts to improve the degree of parental supervision and the overall quality of parenting, since to some extent this disorder may involve a form of self-stimulating behavior. If the parents show sufficient ego strength, some type of behavior modification program may prove to be helpful.

The majority of these patients are probably seen by pediatricians. Those referred to psychiatrists are much more likely to have the associated severe emotional disorders, eliminating Pica as the primary diagnostic category.

307.53   Rumination Disorder of Infancy

This is a rare disorder, more commonly seen by pediatricians than by psychiatrists. Medical causes, such as pyloric stenosis, should be ruled out before a functional etiology is assumed and treated by a psychiatrist. In some respects this appears to be a variant of a "failure to thrive" syndrome. Often hospital admission is required to assess the child's response to feeding in a different environment. The treatment of Rumination Disorder is similar in some respects to that of bulimia in adolescents and young adults. It is important to establish more normal eating patterns, which can be achieved in part through frequent small feedings. This prevents distention and the subsequent need to vomit which may follow the ingestion of a large amount of food by a child who is actually almost starving. The addition of very low doses of antiemetic medication, such as prochlorperazine, may also prove to be helpful.

If the child responds rapidly to a change in environment and caretaker, a careful family assessment should be made, with special attention to the primary caretaker. It may be necessary to treat a parent or other caretaker for problems interfering with the nurturing and bonding process during feeding. Foster care may be necessary in cases of severe family pathology.

307.50   Atypical Eating Disorder

This category is reserved for functional eating disorders that cannot be classified above. It is extremely rare to see a disorder that is completely different from any of those already outlined. The author would therefore recommend that treatment initially follow the guidelines for the disorder it most closely resembles. It should also be noted that unusual or atypical eating disorders are likely to have a medical cause rather than a functional basis.

STEREOTYPED MOVEMENT DISORDERS

DSM-III grades Stereotyped Movement Disorders by increasing severity and duration. There may be different etiologies for these, and different treatment strategies may be suggested; however, the apparent continuum between Transient Tic Disorder and Tourette's Disorder provides for a number of treatment similarities.

307.21   Transient Tic Disorder

Almost all patients with Tourette's Disorder initially meet criteria for Transient Tic Disorder. The treatment for the subgroup who go on to develop signs of Tourette's is much as described in the next section. In a Transient Tic Disorder, psychogenic etiology is likely; however, if there is a family history of tics, a nonpsychogenic cause is very probable.

Transient tics are often mild enough not to require drugs, even though some may be physiologically based. Mild tics usually occur or are exacerbated when the child is under sustained stress, but may improve temporarily with brief stress. Psychotherapy, as indicated by the underlying cause or situational stressor, is recommended.

Patients should be carefully watched for worsening of the tic, social problems or ridicule, and development of other neurologic signs or symptoms.

307.22   Chronic Motor Tic Disorder
307.23   Tourette's Disorder
307.20   Atypical Tic Disorder

Chronic Motor Tic Disorder, Tourette's Disorder, and Atypical Tic Disorder are probably all manifestations of a similar disease process. At this time treatment approaches are essentially the same. I will therefore collectively refer to this group as having Tourette's syndrome.

Many patients who meet the criteria for Chronic Tic Disorder will require medical intervention; almost all patients who meet the criteria for Tourette's Disorder will need some kind of medical help. It is extremely unlikely that either Chronic Motor Tic Disorder or Tourette's Disorder has a primarily psychogenic cause, although life events or the physiologic expression of internal conflict can be at least a partial cause of the symptom fluctuation that typifies these disorders. Patients who have a familial predisposition appear more likely to respond to pharmacologic interventions aimed at altering neurotransmitter balance than do those with no such history.

Approximately 25% of patients with Tourette's syndrome will have an almost total remission when placed on an appropriate dose of haloperidol. This may be as low as 0.5 mg per day, and rarely exceeds 6–8 mg per day. There may be a very narrow therapeutic range of medication for the individual patient, and excessive doses may result in iatrogenic syndromes which resemble Attention Deficit Disorder (including disinhibited behavior and learning disabilities). These may occur in the absence of extrapyramidal side effects and before complete positive response is attained.

About 50% of patients will have considerable, but not total, relief on the above regimen. This is often sufficient for positive social change, with decreased teasing from others and more confidence that embarrassing vocalizations or movements will not occur. Patients who do not improve should have their medication dose decreased without delay. Individual, family, and social interventions other than the medication may also help the patient deal with his or her illness.

Tardive dyskinesia, whose symptoms may be quite similar to those of the tic disorder, is a long-term risk in the use of haloperidol. The clinician must be familiar with this and other risks and with ways of minimizing their potential for occurrence.

For those patients who do not respond to haloperidol, a few other approaches are available. None of these is widely accepted as a treatment of choice, but a trial of each is worthwhile for the refractory patient. Some respond to clonidine, 0.1 to 0.2 mg. Common side effects of clonidine include irritability and hypotension.

A few authorities advocate diet and nutritional approaches as an adjunct to the above treatments. Dietary changes alone may be sufficient to manage milder cases; in others they may lower the required dosage of haloperidol. There appears to be a subgroup of patients whose tics become worse during periods of serotonin deficiency. This may occur one-to-two days after high tryptophan intake, much like a rebound phenomenon. For these patients mild exacerbation can be prevented by having the child avoid meals high in tryptophan. In addition to controlling tryptophan, some authors have recommended supplemental vitamin B-6 and niacinamide in relatively low doses, both of which are said to facilitate the production of serotonin.

In addition to helping the patient deal with feelings about his or her illness, family members should be counseled with regard to the physiologic aspect of the disorder and the fact that although the child can temporarily stop his symptoms, he is not capable of long-term control. The family must understand the relationship between stress and activity and exacerbation of the tics. This should include a discussion of symptoms which may either improve or become worse under acute stress, become worse when stress has just been reduced, or become worse during times when the child must inhibit motor activity while concentrating intensely. The structuring of school and leisure activities to allow discharge of tension often contributes to greater symptom relief from the above treatment approaches.

307.30   Atypical Stereotyped Movement Disorder

This disorder often consists of complex activity such as head-banging, hand-flapping, and the like which is related to severe psychiatric disorder or mental retardation. These activities may simply represent primitive behavior aimed at self-stimulation. Some stereotypic behaviors, however, are a manifestation of dopamine overload which will respond to dopamine blockers such as haloperidol. When medication does not provide significant relief without unacceptable side effects, then carefully constructed behavioral modification programs should be used to interrupt the most troublesome movements. If the patient's disorder endangers him- or herself or others (e.g., head-banging), some sort of protection or restraint may be necessary.

OTHER DISORDERS WITH PHYSICAL MANIFESTATIONS

307.00   Stuttering

Many stutterers do not come to the attention of a psychiatrist, although one may be asked for advice by parents or colleagues. Simple stuttering should not be particularly called to the child's attention during the early stages (when the child is between two and four years old); the best recommendation may be that parents patiently wait for the problem to resolve itself and avoid placing pressure on the child to speed up his or her communication. In a small minority of children, the problem will persist and may become part of a vicious cycle of stuttering, teasing by peers, avoidance of verbal activities in school and social settings, and increased worry about speech.

Medications are generally not indicated. The author has seen some patients who appeared to worsen with low doses of neuroleptics and a few who improved slightly with stimulant or antidepressant medications which were given for other conditions.

Psychotherapy alone does not help most stutterers. When it is used, treatment should focus on helping the patient cope with teasing, low self-esteem, and associated anxiety and depression.

Speech therapists should be called upon for patients with chronic or severe stuttering. Behavioral and learning approaches have a high rate of success when provided by qualified people in the field. Assistance from electrical devices such as those which change auditory biofeedback are recommended by many for the shaping of normal speech habits.

307.60   Functional Enuresis

Patients with Functional Enuresis may be subcategorized into one of several groups. Accurate diagnosis is important, since treatments of choice differ among subgroups.

The most common type of enuresis occurs during deep non-REM sleep. These patients may have a family history of enuresis, and may have associated Sleep Terror Disorder or Sleepwalking Disorder (q.v.). This form of the disorder is quite unresponsive to coercion and behavioral techniques and appears to be well outside the child's volition. Patients often sleep very deeply, and may be known for being difficult to arouse once asleep. Temporary improvement may occur when the child is in a strange bed or sleeping less deeply than usual. Members of this subgroup frequently respond to imipramine. Doses for preschool children may be as low as 10 mg per night; 25 mg per night is more common for six-to-eight-year-olds; higher doses are rarely necessary. Many months or years of drug treatment may be required, but it is often possible to discontinue imipramine after several months. It should be noted that excessive doses of this medication may cause nightmares or other symptoms.

In anxious children for whom imipramine is poorly tolerated, one might consider a milk-free diet with magnesium and calcium supplements. Although relief in many cases is anecdotally documented, the mechanism is not clear. If there is still no response, the parents should be reassured of the child's inability to control the disorder him- or herself, and the high probability that the disorder will be outgrown should be stressed.

A smaller subgroup of enuretic children urinate during REM sleep, often in association with a dream and usually close to the normal awakening time. This form of enuresis is likely to respond well to behavioral techniques, night lights, and simple training devices such as pads which set off an alarm when they become wet. Some of these patients also will respond to a significant reduction in milk intake. Medication is usually not helpful for this group.

Enuresis which can be easily seen as a regressive situational response is treated somewhat differently. The bed-wetting may occur within a state of conscious awareness, most likely close to the time of awakening. The child may awaken and ask for help, perhaps as a way of reassuring him or her that he or she is a focus of love and attention (e.g., soon after the birth of a younger sibling). Psychotherapy with attention to the child's feelings within the family is indicated. Efforts to remove secondary gain, such as having the child help change his or her sheets, having firm expectations that the behavior will cease, and giving reassurance in other parts of family life, may all contribute to a rapid return to age-appropriate behavior.

307.70   Functional Encopresis

Patients with this disorder are more commonly compulsive children from rigid, compulsive families. Emphasis on early control of the bowel and of behaviors and impulses often leads to an inordinate capacity for fecal retention, with occasional episodes of leakage during the day. Patients sometimes respond to a thorough cleansing of an impacted bowel followed by the use of a stool softener or other efforts to improve passage of bowel contents. The emphasis of control then should be shifted, often in a behavioral context, toward encouraging regular bowel movements in an appropriate place; treatment should not focus on simple efforts not to soil.

Family sessions commonly reveal the source of the child's anger and oppositional behavior. There is commonly a very compulsive and controlling mother. This group of children need emphasis on expression of autonomy in more appropriate ways. Family treatment should attempt to alter interpersonal interaction styles.

A second major subtype of Functional Encopresis is that in which the child comes from a severely dissocial and/or dysfunctional family. There has often been little or no effort to train the child. It is not uncommon to have the patient admitted to the hospital, note the considerable attention given by the nursing staff, and have the child be successfully trained by one of the nurses, only to have the problem recur upon his or her return to an unchanged family environment. Social intervention with the family may be very important. Occasionally the level of neglect is so severe that protective agencies must be consulted.

Medication is not generally indicated for Functional Encopresis. Most children gradually gain control of their bowels prior to age eight. The syndrome rarely persists through adolescence.

307.46 Sleepwalking Disorder
Sleepwalking is a problem of deep sleep, most frequently occurring during the third or fourth non-REM stages. The condition is usually self-limited, requiring only reassurance to the parents and efforts to protect the child from injury. Although sleepwalking is rarely an indication of serious psychiatric disorder in children, the family should look for stressors in the child's environment. The symptoms are particularly likely to have to do with the child's fantasied loss of a parent.

In situations in which the sleepwalking is frequent or intractable, simple medical intervention often provides relief. Some children respond to low doses of imipramine. Some studies report that diazepam is helpful for adults; however, there are no controlled studies available in which children were treated in this way.

307.46 Sleep Terror Disorder (307.49)
Sleep terror is another disorder of deep sleep, and is sometimes associated with sleepwalking and a subtype of enuresis. Imipramine has been reported to be helpful; however, true sleep terror should be distinguished from ordinary nightmares before prescribing. During true terrors the child may appear awake but is unresponsive to others and typically has no memory of the episode the next day. Since terrors frequently occur when the child is unusually tired or sleeping very deeply, some authors recommend preventing fatigue and instituting regular schedules of naps and bedtime.

PERVASIVE DEVELOPMENTAL DISORDERS
Because of the long-standing nature of abnormal brain function during critical developmental stages in these children, there is typically considerable distortion in many developmental areas. This makes definitive diagnosis and treatment difficult.

299.0x   Infantile Autism

These severely impaired children may appear intelligent and potentially normal prior to adolescence. The inexperienced clinician may spend many hours in therapy in a futile attempt to reach through the patient's obliviousness to others. Early hopes that intensive psychotherapy would reverse the course of the illness have been disappointing.

Antipsychotic medication has been used in many patients to minimize damage and assist the child in passing through the developmental stages. Neuroleptics have often been disappointing, although a few patients do respond to the potent dopamine-blocking activity of antipsychotics such as haloperidol or fluphenazine. The author has seen a few young patients who improved dramatically with as little as 1–2 mg of haloperidol or fluphenazine per day. It is occasionally necessary to use more sedative medications in patients who are extremely aggressive or self-destructive. Medication is most helpful in adolescent patients.

When the disorder appears to have a primary physiologic or neurotransmitter etiology, there is a greater likelihood that medication will be helpful. More often, the disorder appears more related to temporal lobe damage, in which case behavioral management is more likely to have positive results. A CT scan of the brain can be helpful in making this distinction. Some patients can learn complex vocational skills as they become older. Sign language is commonly used to increase communication with the patient.

There has been some interest in nutritional treatments, either alone or adjunctively. The best documented positive response to these involves high doses of vitamin B-6. There are anecdotal reports of partial improvement in certain patients on milk-free or gluten-free diets. None of these techniques have yet been reported as successful in large controlled studies.

A significant number of patients with Infantile Autism develop severe, explosive temper outbursts in adolescence. This is a common reason for institutionalization after relatively satisfactory progress has been seen in community-based programs for younger patients. The usual neuroleptics are often ineffective for this behavior. Lithium and anticonvulsants have been successful in a limited number of patients.

299.9x   Childhood Onset Pervasive Developmental Disorder

Children with this disorder are less severely impaired than those with Infantile Autism; however, there are some overlapping features. These patients are more likely than autistic children to respond well to medication. The principles just outlined for the biological, behavioral, and educational management of the autistic child generally apply to those with Childhood Onset Pervasive Developmental Disorder. Family and community support groups may assist parents and siblings. Psychotherapy tends to be more helpful for these patients than for the autistic child. The prognosis is poor, but more optimistic than for autism.

299.8x Atypical Pervasive Developmental Disorder
Children with disorders in this residual group should be treated according to presenting symptoms and underlying personal, family, and social factors, using the treatment principles outlined above.

SPECIFIC DEVELOPMENTAL DISORDERS

315.00 Developmental Reading Disorder
A problem of this type often requires the combined efforts of school personnel, psychologist, pediatric neurologist, and child psychiatrist. The child psychiatrist may be more directly involved in treating an associated Conduct Disorder or Attention Deficit Disorder. Modern schools should have programs of individualized instruction and academic intervention based in part on the recommendations made in a complete psychological evaluation. It is rare for children to be treated for this disorder alone. Many "purer" forms are handled entirely within the school system with psychiatric intervention required only because of associated behavioral problems or parental concern.

315.10 Developmental Arithmetic Disorder
This is somewhat more rare than the reading disorder. It is common to see this disorder associated with severe anxiety or incipient thought disorder. Psychiatric treatment should be directed primarily at the associated emotional problems, while allowing school authorities to provide the needed remedial educational programs.

315.31 Developmental Language Disorder
It is important that this diagnosis be made only when the delay in language acquisition is not due to obvious neurologic impairment or mental retardation. It should be distinguished from aphasia since it is the failure to acquire language rather than the loss of language already acquired. Psychiatric intervention in these cases is frequently relatively limited and is likely to involve secondary effects of the problem. For the most part, direct intervention can be most effectively carried out by a speech therapist; however, one may occasionally see a tendency toward improvement with stimulant or antidepressant

medication. Improvement in receptive problems may occur when neuroleptic medications (which may decrease problems of internal distraction) are prescribed.

315.39   Developmental Articulation Disorder

The psychiatrist may be treating the patient for a behavioral problem and find Developmental Articulation Disorder incidentally. The parents should be counseled to seek proper help through a qualified speech therapist.

315.50   Mixed Specific Developmental Disorder

Intervention in these cases frequently involves special education programs within the school, a speech therapist, and psychiatric help to appropriately treat associated emotional problems.

315.90   Atypical Specific Developmental Disorder

Like the above conditions, most of atypical developmental disorders will be treated by school authorities, speech therapists, and the like. The child psychiatrist's involvement should primarily be focused on treating associated behavioral or emotional problems.

Bibliography

MENTAL RETARDATION

Chess, S.: Psychiatric treatment of the mentally retarded child with behavior problems. *American Journal of Orthopsychiatry*, 32:863–869, 1962.

Crandall, B. F.: Genetic counseling and mental retardation. *Psychiatric Annals*, 4(2):70–95, 1974.

Donaldson, J., and Menolascino, F.: Therapeutic and preventive intervention in mental retardation. In G. P. Sholevar, et al. (Eds.), *Treatment of Emotional Disorders in Children and Adolescents*. New York: SP Medical and Scientific Books, 1980, pp. 521–534.

Menolascino, F.: Psychiatric aspects of mental retardation in children under eight. *American Journal of Orthopsychiatry*, 35(5):852–861, 1965.

Menolascino, F. J., and Eaton, L.: Psychoses of childhood: A five-year follow-up study of experiences in a mental retardation clinic. *American Journal of Mental Deficiency*, 72:370–380, 1967.

Nirge, B.: The normalization principle and its human management implications. In R. Kugel and W. Wolfensberger (Eds.), *Changing Patterns in Residential Services for the Mentally Retarded*. Washington: Government Printing Office, 1969.

Pasamanick, B.: Research on the influence of sociocultural variables upon organic factors in mental retardation. *American Journal of Mental Deficiency*, 64:316–322, 1959.

Solnit, A., and Stark, M.: Mourning and the birth of a defective child. *Psychoanalytic Study of the Child*, 16:523–537, 1961.

Webster, T. G.: Unique aspects of emotional development in mentally retarded children. In F. J. Menolascino (Ed.), *Psychiatric Approaches to Mental Retardation*. New York: Basic Books, 1970.

Zigler, E.: Familial mental retardation: A continuing dilemma. *Science*, 155:292–298, 1967.

ATTENTION DEFICIT DISORDER

Cantwell, D. P., and Carlson, G. A.: Stimulants. In J. S. Werry (Ed.), *Pediatric Psychopharmacology: The Use of Behavior Modifying Drugs in Children*. New York: Brunner/Mazel, 1978.

Donaldson, J.: Some considerations in the treatment of hyperactive children. *Nebraska Medical Journal*, 60(6):194–196, 1975.

Eisenberg, L.: Symposium: Behavior modification by drugs. The clinical use of stimulant drugs in children. *Pediatrics,* 49:709-715, 1972.

Feingold, B.: Food additives and child development. *Hospital Practice,* 8:11-12, 17-19, 1973.

Fish, B.: The "one child, one drug" myth of stimulants in hyperkinesis: Importance of diagnostic categories in evaluating treatment. *Archives of General Psychiatry,* 24:193-203, 1971.

Fish, B.: Drug treatment of the hyperactive child. In D. Cantwell (Ed.), *The Hyperactive Child: Diagnosis, Management and Current Research.* New York: Spectrum Publications, 1975, pp. 109-127.

Gardner, R. A.: Psychotherapy of the psychogenic problems secondary to minimal brain dysfunction. *International Journal of Psychotherapy,* 2:224-256, 1973.

Rapoport, J. L., and Mikkelsen, E. J.: Antidepressants. In J. Werry (Ed.), *Pediatric Psychopharmacology: The Use of Behavior Modifying Drugs in Children.* New York: Brunner/Mazel, 1978, pp. 208-233.

Rapoport, J. L., Quin, P. O., Bradbard, G., et al.: Imipramine and methylphenidate treatments of hyperactive boys. *Archives of General Psychiatry,* 30:789-793, 1974.

Satterfield, J. H., Cantwell, D. P., and Satterfield, B. T.: Pathophysiology of the hyperactive child syndrome. *Archives of General Psychiatry,* 31:839-844, 1974.

Schrager, J., Lindy, J., Harrison, S., et al.: The hyperkinetic child: An overview of the issue. *Journal of the American Academy of Child Psychiatry,* 5:526-533, 1966.

Wender, P.: *The Hyperactive Child: A Guide for Parents.* New York: Crown, 1973.

Werry, J. S., Weiss, G., Douglas, V., and Martin, J.: Studies on the hyperactive child. III. The effect of chlorpromazine upon behavior and learning disability. *Journal of the American Academy of Child Psychiatry,* 5:292-312, 1966.

CONDUCT DISORDER

Bender, L. (Ed.): Studies on aggression in children. *Aggression, Hostility and Anxiety in Children,* Springfield, IL: Charles C Thomas, 1953, pp. 3-40.

Cantwell, D. P.: Hyperactivity and antisocial behavior. *Journal of the American Academy of Child Psychiatry,* 17:252-262, 1978.

Eisenberg, L., Lachman, R., Molling, P., et al.: A psychopharmacologic experiment in a training school for delinquent boys: Methods, problems, findings. *American Journal of Orthopsychiatry,* 33:431-447, 1963.

Glueck, S., and Glueck, E.: *Toward a Typology of Juvenile Offenders.* New York: Grune and Stratton, 1970.

Jenkins, R.: Classification of behavior problems of children. *American Journal of Psychiatry,* 125(8):1032, 1969.

Johnson, A. M.: Sanctions for superego lacunae of adolescents. In K. R. Eissler (Ed.), *Searchlights on Delinquency.* New York: International Universities Press, 1949.

Levy, D.: Oppositional syndromes and oppositional behavior. In P. H. Hoch and J. Zubin (Eds.), *Psychopathology of Childhood.* New York: Grune and Stratton, 1955, pp. 204-227.

Mednick, S. A., and Christiansen, K. O. (Eds.): *Biosocial Bases of Criminal Behavior.* New York: Halstead Press, 1977.

Minuchin, S., and Montalvo, B.: Techniques for working with disorganized low socioeconomic families. *American Journal of Orthopsychiatry,* 37:880-887, 1967.

Redl, F.: The concept of a "therapeutic milieu." *American Journal of Orthopsychiatry,* 29:721-736, 1959.

Redl, F., and Wineman, D.: *Controls from Within: Techniques for the Treatment of the Aggressive Child.* New York: Free Press, 1954.

Satterfield, J. H., and Cantwell, D. P.: Psychopharmacology in the prevention of antisocial and delinquent behavior. In R. Gittelman-Klein (Ed.), *Recent Advances in Child Psychopharmacology.* New York: Human Sciences Press, 1975.

Thomas, A., and Chess, S.: Evaluation of behavior disorders into adolescence. *American Journal of Psychiatry*, 133(5), 1976.

ANXIETY DISORDERS OF CHILDHOOD OR ADOLESCENCE

Barcai, A., and Rosenthal, M.: Fears and tyranny. *Archives of General Psychiatry*, 30:392–395, 1974.
Berlin, I. N.: Crisis intervention and short-term therapy: An approach in a child-psychiatric clinic. *American Academy of Child Psychiatry*, 9:595–606, 1970.
Carek, D. J.: *Principles of Child Psychotherapy*. Springfield, IL: Charles C Thomas, 1972.
Eisenberg, L.: Principles of drug therapy in child psychiatry. *American Journal of Orthopsychiatry*, 41(3):311–380, 1970.
English, O., and Pearson, G.: Irrational fears and phobias. *Emotional Problems in Living*, 3rd Edition. New York: W. W. Norton, 1963.
Gittelman-Klein, R., and Klein, D. F.: School phobia: Diagnostic considerations in the light of imipramine effects. *Journal of Nervous and Mental Disease*, 156:199–215, 1973.
Haworth, M. R. (Ed.): *Child Psychotherapy: Practice and Theory*. New York: Basic Books, 1964.
McAndrew, J. B., Case, Q., and Treffert, D. A.: Effects of prolonged phenothiazine intake in psychotic and other hospitalized children. *Journal of Autism and Childhood Schizophrenia*, 2:75–91, 1972.
Minde, K. W., and Weiss, G. D.: The assessment of drug effects in children as compared to adults. *American Academy of Child Psychiatry*, 9:124–133, 1970.
Poznanski, E. O.: Children with excessive fears. *American Journal of Orthopsychiatry*, 43:428–438, 1973.
Sandler, J., and Joffe, W. G.: Notes on obsessional manifestations in children. *Psychoanalytic Study of the Child*, 20:425–438, 1965.
Saraf, K. R., Klein, D. F., Gittelman-Klein, R., and Groff, S.: Imipramine side effects in children. *Psychopharmacologia*, 37(3):265–274, 1974.
Sperling, M.: School phobia: Classification, dynamics and treatment. *Psychoanalytic Study of the Child*, 22:375–401, 1967.
Wahler, R.: Oppositional children: A quest for parental reinforcement control. *Journal of Applied Behavioral Analysis*, 2:159–170, 1969.
Werry, J.: The use of psychotropic drugs in children. *Journal of the American Academy of Child Psychiatry*, 16(3):353–405, 1977.

OTHER DISORDERS OF INFANCY, CHILDHOOD, OR ADOLESCENCE

Adams, P. L.: *Obsessive Children: A Sociopsychiatric Study*. New York: Brunner/Mazel, 1973.
Ainsworth, M.: The development of infant-mother attachment. In B. Caldwell and M. Ricciuti (Eds.), *Child Development Research*, #3. Chicago: University of Chicago Press, 1973, pp. 1–99.
Barcai, A., and Rosenthal, M.: Fears and tyranny. *Archives of General Psychiatry*, 30:392–395, 1974.
Blank, M.: Some maternal influences on infants' rates of sensory-motor development. *Journal of the American Academy of Child Psychiatry*, 3:93–104, 1964.
Bowlby, J.: The nature of a child's tie to his mother. *International Journal of Psychoanalysis*, 39:350–373, 1958.
Elson, A., Pearson, C., et al.: Follow-up study of childhood elective mutism. *Archives of General Psychiatry*, 13:182–187, 1964.
Erikson, E. H.: *Childhood and Society*, 2nd Edition. New York: W. W. Norton, 1963.

Halpern, W. I., Hammond, J., and Cohen, R.: A therapeutic approach to speech phobia: Elective mutism reexamined. *Journal of the American Academy of Child Psychiatry*, 10:94–107, 1971.

Hayden, T. L.: Classification of elective mutism. *Journal of the American Academy of Child Psychiatry*, 19:118–133, 1980.

Levy, D.: Oppositional syndromes and oppositional behavior. In P. H. Hoch and J. Zubin (Eds.), *Psychopathology of Childhood*. New York: Grune and Stratton, 1955, pp. 204–227.

Rutter, M.: Maternal deprivation, 1972–1978—New findings, new concepts, new approaches. *Child Development*, 50(2):283–305, 1979.

Wahler, R.: Oppositional children: A quest for parental reinforcement control. *Journal of Applied Behavior Analysis*, 2:159–170, 1969.

EATING DISORDERS

Agras, W. S., Barlow, D. H., Chapin, H. N., et al.: Behavior modification of anorexia nervosa. *Archives of General Psychiatry*, 30:279–286, 1974.

Bruch, H.: Perils of behavior modification in treatment of anorexia nervosa. *Journal of the American Medical Association*, 230:1419–1422, 1974.

Bruch, H.: *The Golden Cage: The Enigma of Anorexia Nervosa*. Cambridge, MA: Harvard University Press, 1978.

Escalona, S.: Feeding disturbances in very young children. *American Journal of Orthopsychiatry*, 15:76–80, 1945.

Flanagan, C. H.: Rumination in infancy—past and present. With a case report. *Journal of the American Academy of Child Psychiatry*, 16(1):140–149, 1977.

Garfinkel, P. E., and Garner, D. M. *Anorexia Nervosa: A Multidimensional Perspective*. New York: Brunner/Mazel, 1982.

Gull, W. W.: Anorexia nervosa. *Trans. Clin. Soc.* (London), 7:22–28 (1874). Reprinted in S. I. Harrison and J. F. McDermott (Eds.), *Childhood Psychopathology: An Anthology of Basic Readings*. New York: International Universities Press, 1972.

Hoyt, C. S., and Stickler, G. B.: A study of 44 children with the syndrome of recurrent (cyclic) vomiting. *Pediatrics*, 25:775–780, 1960.

Lang, P. J., and Melamed, B. G.: Case report: Avoidance conditioning therapy of an infant with chronic ruminative vomiting. *Journal of Abnormal Psychology*, 74(1):1–8, 1969.

Levenkron, S.: *The Best Little Girl in the World*. New York: Contemporary Books, 1978.

Liebman, R., Minuchin, S., and Baker, L.: The role of the family in the treatment of anorexia nervosa. *Journal of Child Psychiatry*, 13:264–274, 1974.

Manningo, F. V., and Delgado, R. A.: Trichotillomania in children: A review. *American Journal of Psychiatry*, 26:505–511, 1969.

Maxmen, J. S., Siberfarb, P. M., and Ferrell, R. B.: Anorexia nervosa: Practical initial management in a general hospital. *Journal of the American Medical Association*, 229(7):801–803, 1974.

Russell, G.: Bulimia nervosa: An ominous variant of anorexia nervosa. *Psychological Medicine*, 9:429–448, 1979.

STEREOTYPED MOVEMENT DISORDERS

Cohen, D. J., and Young, J. G.: Neurochemistry and child psychiatry. *Journal of the American Academy of Child Psychiatry*, 16:353–411, 1977.

Golden, G. S.: Tics and Tourette's: A continuum of symptoms? *Annals of Neurology*, 2(3): 260, 1977.

Lowe, T. L., Cohen, D. J., Detlor, J., Kremenitzer, M. W., and Shaywitz, B. A.: Stimulant medications precipitate Tourette's syndrome. *Journal of the American Medical Association*, 247(12):1729–1731, 1982.

McKeith, I. G., Williams, A., and Nicol, A. R.: Clonidine in Tourette syndrome, *Lancet*, January 31, 1981, pp. 270–271.

Mitchell, E., and Matthews, K. L.: Gilles de la Tourette's disorder associated with pemoline. *American Journal of Psychiatry*, 137(12):1618–1619, December 1980.

Shapiro, A. K., Shapiro, E., and Wayne, H. L.: The symptomatology and diagnosis of Tourette's syndrome. *Journal of the American Academy of Child Psychiatry*, 12(4):702–723, 1973.

Singer, H. S., Butler, I., Seifert, W., Caprioli, R., and Koslow, S.: Tourette syndrome: A neurotransmitter disorder? *Annals of Neurology*, 4(2):189–190, 1978.

Snyder, S. H., Banerjee, S. P., Yamamura, H. I., and Greenberg, D.: Drugs, neurotransmitters and schizophrenia. *Science*, 184:1243–1253, 1974.

Tanner, C. M., Goetz, C. G., and Klawans, H. L.: Cholinergic and anticholinergic effects in Tourette syndrome. *Neurology*, 30(4):384, 1980.

Woodrow, K. M. Gilles de la Tourette's disease: A review. *American Journal of Psychiatry*, 131: 100–103, 1974.

OTHER DISORDERS WITH PHYSICAL MANIFESTATIONS

Anders, T., and Weinstein, P.: Sleep and its disorders in infants and children (Review). *Journal of Pediatrics*, 50(2):311–324, 1972.

Anthony, E. J.: An experimental approach to the psychopathology: Encopresis. In S. I. Harrison and J. F. McDermott (Eds.), *Childhood Psychopathology: An Anthology of Basic Readings*. New York: International Universities Press, 1972, pp. 610–625.

Beech, H., and Fransella, F.: *Research and Experiments in Stuttering*. Oxford, England: Pergamon Press, 1968.

Esman, A.: Nocturnal enuresis: Some current concepts. *Journal of the American Academy of Child Psychiatry*, 16(1):150–158, Winter 1977.

Fisher, S. M.: Encopresis. In J. D. Noshpitz (Ed.), *Basic Handbook of Child Psychiatry*, Volume 2. New York: Basic Books, 1979, pp. 556–568.

Fraiberg, S.: On the sleep disturbances of early childhood. *Childhood Psychopathology: An Anthology of Basic Readings*, 1972, 310–339.

Halpern, W.: The treatment of encopretic children. *Journal of the American Academy of Child Psychiatry*, 16:478–499, 1977.

Ragins, N., and Schacter, J.: A study of sleep behavior in two-year-old children. *Journal of the American Academy of Child Psychiatry*, 10:464–489, 1971.

Ryan, B. P.: *Programmed Therapy for Stuttering in Children and Adults*. Springfield, IL: Charles C Thomas, 1974.

Shames, G.: Dysfluency and stuttering. *Pediatric Clinics of North America*, 15:691, 1968.

PERVASIVE DEVELOPMENTAL DISORDERS

Bender, L.: Childhood Schizophrenia. *American Journal of Orthopsychiatry*, 17:40–57, 1947.

Cohen, D., and Young, G.: Neurochemistry in child psychiatry. *Journal of the American Academy of Child Psychiatry*, 10(3):353–405, 1977.

Eisenberg, L.: Principles of drug therapy in child psychiatry. *American Journal of Orthopsychiatry*, 41(3):311–380, April, 1970.

Fish, B.: Neurobiologic antecedents of schizophrenia in children, *Archives of General Psychiatry*, 34:1297–1313, 1977.

Fish, B., and Ritvo, E. R.: Psychoses of childhood. In J. D. Noshpitz (Ed.), *Basic Handbook of Child Psychiatry*, Volume 2. New York: Basic Books, 1979, pp. 249–303.

Goldfarb, W.: An investigation of childhood schizophrenia: Retrospective view. *Archives of General Psychiatry*, 11:620–634, 1969.

Kanner, L., and Lesser, L.: Early infantile autism. *Pediatric Clinics of North America*, 5(3):711–730, 1958.

Mahler, M.: On childhood psychosis and schizophrenia: Autistic and symbiotic infantile psychosis. *Psychoanalytic Study of the Child*, 7:286–305, 1952.

Ornitz, E. M., and Ritvo, E. R.: The syndrome of autism: A critical review. *American Journal of Psychiatry*, 133(6):609–621, 1976.

Rutter, M.: The development of infantile autism. *Psychological Medicine*, 4:147–163, 1974.

Werry, J.: The use of psychotropic drugs in children. *Journal of the American Academy of Child Psychiatry*, 16(3):353–405, 1977.

SPECIFIC DEVELOPMENTAL DISORDERS

Buxbaum, E.: The parent's role in the etiology of learning disabilities. *Psychoanalytic Study of the Child*, 19, 1964.

Mattis, S., French, J. H., and Rapin, I.: Dyslexia in children and young adults. In S. Chess and A. Thomas (Eds.), *Annual Progress in Child Psychiatry and Child Development*, 1976. New York: Brunner/Mazel, 1977.

Rutter, M.: Emotional disorder and educational underachievement. *Archives of Disease in Childhood*, 49:249–256, 1974.

Silver, A., and Hagin, R.: Specific reading disability: Follow-up studies. *American Journal of Orthopsychiatry*, 34:95–102, 1964.

Section II

by

George U. Balis, M.D.

Chapter 2

Organic Mental Disorders

The format for Section II differs somewhat from that of the remainder of this book. While an effort has been made to follow the DSM-III outline of psychiatric disorders exactly, such a format would be unwieldly when addressing the treatment of Organic Mental Disorders. We have accordingly grouped the disorders in a clinically useful way—much as DSM-III provides early in its section on Organic Mental Disorders.

For those readers who wish to locate specific diagnostic codes, the following table of contents is provided:

Substance-induced Organic Mental Disorders

Alcohol Organic Mental Disorders

Barbiturate or Similarly Acting Sedative or Hypnotic Organic Mental Disorders

Opioid Organic Mental Disorders

Cocaine Organic Mental Disorder

Amphetamine or Similarly Acting Sympathomimetic Organic Mental Disorders

**Organic Mental Disorders in which the etiology or pathophysiological
process is either noted as an additional diagnosis from outside of the
mental disorders section of ICD-9-CM (Axis III) or is unknown**

DEFINITION
Organic Mental Disorders are a category of disorders manifesting disturbances of mental functioning and behavior that result from known or presumed damage or dysfunction of the brain. The term *Organic Brain Syndromes* is used to refer to characteristic constellations of signs and symptoms that result from damage or dysfunction of the brain without making reference to the underlying specific etiology. The former constitutes an etiological diagnosis, while the latter constitutes a syndromatic diagnosis. It is the etiological diagnosis that upgrades a syndrome into a disorder and allows for specific treatment.

GENERAL PRINCIPLES OF TREATMENT AND PATIENT MANAGEMENT
The therapeutic approach to the patient with an Organic Mental Disorder is based on a truly biopsychosocial model. Although a biomedical understanding of the underlying disease process is of primary importance, an understanding of the psychosocial aspects of the illness is also of major importance in the treatment and management of these patients (Stern, 1982).

The therapeutic approach to these patients can be divided into (a) treatment and (b) patient management. Those approaches that utilize specific medical procedures (e.g., drug therapy, surgery, psychotherapy) are referred to as *treatment*. Treatment is further distinguished into *etiological* and *symptomatic*, on the basis of whether the therapeutic method aims at eliminating the cause of the disease or merely removing or improving its symptoms. All the nonspecific interventions which are part of the therapeutic effort are referred to as *management* and are generally supportive in nature.

Treatment
The *etiological treatment*, when such treatment is available, is clearly of overriding significance, since it aims at removing the cause of the disorder and allowing the reparative process to correct the underlying pathology. It is

imperative, therefore, that every effort be made to identify and treat the underlying disorder by eliminating its cause, and correcting its consequences, whenever possible. When etiological treatment is unavailable or the cause of the disorder is still unknown, one is limited to the use of symptomatic treatment.

The *symptomatic treatment* is directed toward two areas: (a) the removal or control of the physical symptoms of the underlying disorder and the normalization of physiological functioning in all systems affected by the disease process; and (b) the removal or control of psychopathology associated with the OBS, through the use of various psychiatric treatment modalities which include both pharmacologic and psychosocial approaches. Furthermore, the psychiatric treatment is also directed at restoring the patient's psychosocial functioning to the extent that this is possible, and at improving his or her adjustment to residual cognitive deficits.

Patient Management

Medicine is not only an applied scientific discipline, but also an art that involves the skillful application of management principles as an integral part of treatment. Patient management is a very important aspect of the total effort to provide comprehensive care that meets the current and anticipated needs of the patient and his family. Management interventions aim at reducing morbidity, increasing comfort through relief of suffering, enhancing impaired functions, increasing available competence skills, reducing the need for lost functions, and generally optimizing the patient's psychosocial milieu, including his or her physical environment, family, and social setting. The effectiveness of the clinician in patient management depends on:

(a) knowledge of the underlying pathogenic mechanisms responsible for the physiological and psychological disturbances of the syndrome and the way these disturbances impact upon the patient's personality and behavior;

(b) understanding of the patient's personality and, in the face of stress, loss of function, and loss of self-esteem;

(c) sensitivity to patient needs and empathic caring in meeting these needs;

(d) ability to utilize available resources within the hospital, the patient's family, and his/her community in the effort to treat and rehabilitate him or her; and

(e) ability to work cooperatively with other health professionals, independently or within a team approach.

Depending on the type of Organic Brain Syndrome (e.g., Delirium, Dementia), different management approaches must be applied within different settings and varying circumstances. Effective approaches vary according to whether the patient is managed in the emergency room, medical-surgical ward or I.C.U., his or her own home, the physician's office, or a nursing home. The appropriate locus of treatment is determined by the type of care the patient needs, i.e., acute care settings (general hospital or psychiatric unit) for the acutely disturbed, physically ill, delirious, psychotic, or depressed patient; intermediate care or chronic care settings (nursing homes, half-way houses) for patients with protracted or chronic syndromes requiring a lower level of care, or a sheltered or structured environment; or a home care setting for those who can be managed at home and in the physician's office. The patient's need for particular management skills and interventions may vary during the stages of the clinical course of the syndrome (e.g., acute phase, convalescence, or chronic), as well as according to the prognosis of the syndrome (reversible or irreversible, static or progressive). The primary physician must be thoroughly familiar with the management of the delirious patient in a hospital setting (Dubovsky & Weisberg, 1982).

Of particular significance is the management of patients with chronic impairment, Dementia, Organic Amnestic Syndrome, and Organic Personality Syndrome. These patients require continuous management efforts that aim at reducing need for impaired or lost function and maximizing utilization of available function, as well as preventing regression, dependency, and other reactive psychopathology. The management of those patients who suffer from OBS associated with minimal or no cognitive deficit (Organic Hallucinosis, Organic Delusional Syndrome, and Organic Affective Syndrome) is similar to that of patients with the corresponding functional disorders.

The management of patients whose OBS is secondary to substance abuse is of great importance, especially during the period following recovery from the syndrome. Follow-up treatment and rehabilitation for substance abuse represent an indispensable part of the total therapeutic management.

Finally, the family of the patient, his or her home environment, and the social milieu are, in most instances, a major focus in the effort for effective management. Counseling with family members, especially spouse or primary caretakers, may involve a range of concerns, including advice regarding the care and supervision of the patient, reducing stress and resolving conflict within the family, dealing with unrealistic expectations about prognosis of current and future capacity to function, and assisting family members in effective coping strategies, especially in caring for the chronically demented, psychotic, or impulsive and emotionally unstable person.

DELIRIA
Almost every one of the causes of Organic Mental Disorders listed in Table 1 may result in delirium, acting alone or in combination with several other factors (multifactorial etiology). Its most common etiology involves drug intoxication or idiosyncrasy, or withdrawal from alcohol or hypnotic-sedative drugs. Various metabolic disorders, infectious diseases, endocrinopathies, systemic disorders, and primary CNS disorders (including infections, head trauma, postictal syndromes, neoplasms, and cerebrovascular disorders) are also relatively common.

General Therapeutic Principles
The treatment and management of the delirious patient are generally based upon the following therapeutic principles:

(a) Identify and treat the causative factor(s) of the underlying primary disorder;

(b) Understand the pathogenic mechanisms of the disease process that led to the development of the delirium;

(c) Recognize emergency situations for early treatment intervention in order to prevent the possibility of irreversible brain damage or death (e.g., anoxia, hypoglycemia);

(d) Recognize and treat those psychiatric symptoms that must be removed in order to provide relief or prevent accidents or complications (e.g., agitation, combativeness, suicidal behavior); and

(e) Understand the particular cognitive state of the delirious patient and factors that may influence it, in order to optimize nonspecific supportive measures in patient management (e.g., impaired capacity for information processing as influenced by an unfamiliar or ambiguous environment) (Balis, 1970; Sakles & Balis, 1978).

Etiologic Treatment
Every effort should be made to identify the underlying causative factor(s) with the aim of instituting specific treatment at the earliest possible time. A detailed history from relatives or friends is most helpful, especially in identifying drug ingestion, alcohol abuse, head trauma, chemical exposure, or already diagnosed disease (e.g., diabetes, epilepsy, drug idiosyncrasies, or heart disease). In hospitalized patients, the diagnostic process is aided by focusing on the setting in which the delirium occurred (I.C.U., recovery room, dialysis unit), the nature of preexisting disease (e.g., pulmonary insufficiency, cardiac failure, hepatic cirrhosis), or the nature of treatment of the primary

TABLE 1
Causes of Organic Mental Disorders

Intracranial Infections	Epidemic encephalitis (arthropod borne, entero-viruses, lethargica); sporadic encephalitis (herpes simplex, mumps, herpes zoster, infectious hepatitis, rabies); post-infectious encephalitis (influenza, measles, rubella, post-vaccination, chickenpox, scarlet fever, atypical pneumonia, infectious mononucleosis); subacute-chronic encephalitis (Dawson's subacute inclusion body, Von Bogaert's subacute sclerosing leukoencephalitis, subacute sclerosing panencephalitis, Creutzfeldt-Jakob disease, progressive multifocal leukoencephalopathy, kuru); neurosyphilis (meningovascular, general paresis); cerebral abscess; meningitis.
Degenerative	Alzheimer's senile-presenile dementia, Pick's disease, Huntington's chorea, Parkinson's disease, progressive supranuclear palsy, simple cortical atrophy.
Vascular	Thrombosis, embolism, intracerebral and subarachnoid embolism, temporal arteritis, migraine, multi-infarct dementia, carotid artery occlusal disease, Binswanger's disease.
Cerebral Injury	Head trauma, radiation, hyperthermia, electric current.
Space-occupying Lesions	Neoplasms, subdural hematoma, aneurysms, colloid cyst, parasitic cyst, tuberculoma, lymphoma.
Epilepsy	Postictal syndromes, epileptic personality, epileptic dementia, epileptic psychosis, psychomotor seizures.
Other CNS Disorders	Multiple sclerosis, normal pressure hydrocephalus, Tourette's syndrome, narcolepsy, Schilder's disease.

TABLE 1 *(continued)*

Substances	Alcohol, anticholinergic drugs, sedative-hypnotics, hallucinogens, opiates, sympathomimetic stimulants, cannabis, phencyclidine or arylcyclohexylamines, antihypertensive drugs, antiarrhythmic drugs, digitalis, cimetidine, anticonvulsants, steroids, etc.
Poisons/ Chemicals	Heavy metals (lead, mercury, arsenic, thalium); industrial poisons (carbon monoxide and disulfide, organic solvents, methylchloride).
Systemic Infections	Pneumonia, typhoid, typhus, acute rheumatic fever, malaria, diphtheria, Legionnaires' disease, brucellosis, Rocky Mountain spotted fever.
Systemic Disease Affecting CNS	Systemic lupus erythematosus, hypertensive encephalopathy, rheumatoid vasculitis, polyarteritis nodosa, Sydenham's chorea, porphyria, Paget's disease, Wilson's disease.
Metabolic Diseases	Diabetic acidosis or hypoglycemia; hepatic, renal, and pulmonary insufficiency or failure; dialysis dementia, jejunoileostomy psychosis.
Electrolytes/ Water	Hypo- or hyper-calcemia, hypo- or hyper-natremia, hypo- or hyper-kalemia, dehydration, overhydration, acid-base disturbance.
Blood Gases	Hypoxia-anoxia, due to cardiac disease, shock, anemia, pulmonary disease.
Endocrinopathies	Hypo- or hyper-thyroidism, hyperparathyroidism, Cushing's syndrome, Addison's disease, hypopituitarism, hyperinsulinism.
Vitamin Deficiencies	Nicotinic acid (pellagra), thiamine (Korsakoff-Wernicke), B12 and folate (pernicious anemia), A and D hypervitaminosis.
Miscellaneous	Total sleep deprivation, sarcoidosis, carcinoid syndrome, pheochromocytoma, remote effects of CA, serum sickness, sensory isolation, severe burns, food allergy.

disorder (e.g., digitalization, hypnotic-sedatives, continuous gastric suction, irradiation).

In view of the fact that the etiology of delirium is often multifactorial, especially in the hospitalized patient, the clinician should make an effort to search for several possible causative factors rather than a singular etiology. Although a single factor may cause delirium, several subthreshold factors acting concurrently may be necessary to produce the critical derangement of "cerebral insufficiency" that leads to the decompensated state. In this regard, every pathophysiological abnormality should be corrected and every possible etiologic factor eliminated, especially nonessential medications or those for which a less toxic drug can be substituted.

Once the causative factor is removed, the condition may be self-limited with rapid and complete recovery. In some instances, the primary cause may have already ceased to operate (e.g., head trauma, burns, seizures, bleeding, radiation) and only the pathogenic sequelae need to be treated (secondary causes). In other instances, the primary cause is unknown and only the disease processes are identifiable and amenable to treatment (e.g., effects of unknown drugs, fever of unknown origin). Sometimes all efforts fail to provide evidence of "organic" factors which seem related to a clinical delirium.

While searching for an etiologic diagnosis of the delirium, the clinician is called upon to recognize emergency situations presenting with delirium, either because they may be life-threatening or because of the possibility of irreversible brain damage (dementia) should the condition be prolonged. Early recognition and emergency treatment intervention reduce risk or degree of brain injury, as well as general morbidity and mortality risk. Common preventable etiologies associated with such risk include drug intoxication, hypoglycemia, diabetic acidosis, hypoxia or anoxia, thiamine deficiency, intracranial hemorrhage, subdural hematoma, subarachnoid or intracerebral hemorrhage due to ruptured aneurysm, withdrawal delirium, acute cerebral edema, and hyperthermia. Delirium as a complication of a serious illness may often serve as a prognostic criterion of life-threatening or ominous outcome.

Symptomatic Treatment

This is directed toward two areas: psychiatric symptoms of the delirium, and the physical symptoms of the underlying disorder. Its purpose is to provide relief, improve morbidity, and prevent complications through an appropriately targeted approach to symptom control. Symptomatic treatment may be the only therapeutic approach available in those instances in which etiologic diagnosis is lacking.

The symptomatic treatment of the delirium is primarly medicinal. It should be emphasized, however, that the clinical picture of many delirious patients may not require any medical treatment other than general supportive management, and that appropriate management approaches may minimize or make unnecessary the use of drug treatment. For instance, when the clinical picture is characterized by a simple confusional state without symptoms of agitation, fear, or combativeness, medicinal treatment is unnecessary and may even be contraindicated since the psychotropic drugs that are commonly used for symptomatic relief may aggravate the delirium through their depressant, anticholinergic, or hypotensive effects (Heizer & Wilbert, 1974). Even in florid deliria in which the patient's emotional and behavioral reaction to the cognitive impairment dominates the clinical picture, pharmacologic control of symptoms should be judicious and tempered by the realization that appropriately supportive management measures may be of equal or even of greater importance.

Medicinal control of delirium generally involves the relief of distressing symptoms (fear, anxiety, panic, irritability, angry outbursts, illusory and hallucinatory symptoms, delusions) and disruptive behaviors (excitement, agitation, restlessness, combativeness, assaultiveness, hyperactivity, insomnia). Psychotropic drugs have no therapeutic effect on the cognitive deficit, and as mentioned earlier, may even worsen it. Physostigmine will restore cognitive functions in deliria induced by anticholinergic agents. Drugs recommended for the *symptomatic* control of delirious symptoms include neuroleptics (antipsychotic drugs), antianxiety drugs (benzodiazepines and antihistamines), and hypnotics. The choice of a particular psychotropic drug is based on several considerations, including etiology of the delirium, biometabolism and side effects of the drug, and one's previous experience. Thorough familiarity with a drug's pharmacological actions, pharmacokinetics, biometabolism, and side effects enables the physician to tailor the treatment to the patient's particular needs.

High potency neuroleptics (haloperidol, perphenazine, thiothixene, fluphenazine, and trifluoperazine) show minimal sedative and autonomic (anticholinergic and alpha-blocking) effects, but a high incidence of extrapyramidal reactions (dystonias and parkinsonism). They are effective in the control of the delirious psychopathology including agitation, fear, and psychotic symptoms. The neuroleptic of choice in most cases is haloperidol (Haldol) (Ayd, 1978).

The anxiolytic benzodiazepines (chlordiazepoxide, diazepam, oxazepam, etc.) are safe and effective. They are less sedating than the hypnotics, require high doses to produce CNS depression, and have minimal autonomic action or effect on the cardiovascular and respiratory systems. They have a measurable anticonvulsant activity that may be useful in treating withdrawal deliria. They differ in pharmacokinetics and biometabolism, with oxazepam having a short plasma half-life, and chlordiazepoxide and diazepam lasting much longer. Oxazepam may therefore be the benzodiazepine of choice for treating patients expected to show cumulative effects (hepatic or renal insufficiency or prolonged use of the drug) (Lipowski, 1980a, b).

The prescription schedule of any of these drugs should also take into consideration the fluctuating course of delirium. If the timing of occurrence of the symptoms is characteristic (e.g., at night), it is advisable to prescribe the drug only just prior to the onset of symptoms (Dubovsky & Weisberg, 1982).

The dosage and route of administration of these drugs depend on the severity of the symptoms, responsiveness to the drug, the patient's age (the elderly require much lower doses), and other factors. Small, preferably oral dosages are appropriate for moderate anxiety and restlessness. Higher doses, given parenterally, are required for the control of severe agitation, panic states, or assaultive behavior. The art of optimal titration of the drug, in order to be able to meet the changing needs of the delirious patient, requires close monitoring of therapeutic response and knowledge of all factors that may modify drug effects. Common problems associated with a failure to titrate the drug optimally include *oversedation* ("snowing" effect) resulting in stupor or even coma and respiratory depression, or *undersedation* with ineffective control of the symptoms.

When the choice of drug is haloperidol, the following approach is generally recommended. In mildly to moderately agitated patients, 2–10 mg given orally twice a day generally suffice. Parenteral administration might be necessary for the uncooperative patient, with the dosage adjusted about three-fourths of the oral amount. In severely agitated, assaultive, or panicked patients, haloperidol should be given parenterally (I.M.), with an initial dose of 2–10 mg, which can be repeated several times a day as needed, until control of agitation is achieved (Lipowski, 1980a, b). The so-called "rapid neuroleptization method" has been suggested as a means of handling emergency situations and is described on page 113. Doses should be lower than those for non-organic disorders. The total daily dose required to produce a calming effect may range from 10–40 mg (or higher). Once this effect is achieved the haloperidol should be given orally, in b.i.d. doses (Moore, 1977), and be gradually tapered off and discontinued within days or weeks.

When benzodiazepines are used, the choice depends primarily on differences in their plasma half-lives and hepatic metabolism. In mildly to moderately agitated patients, 25–30 mg of chlordiazepoxide, 5–10 mg of diazepam, or 15–30 mg of oxazepam, given orally every four to six hours as needed, is generally sufficient. These doses may be doubled in more severely agitated patients. Parenteral administration of chlordiazepoxide may be required for patients showing severe agitation, panic, or combativeness, at dosage levels comparable to those for oral administration. In emergency situations, slow intravenous injection of chlordiazepoxide (25–50 mg) or diazepam (5–10 mg) may become necessary in order to bring the symptoms under immediate control.

Hydroxyzine, an antihistamine, and paraldehyde, a hypnotic, may also be used for control of anxiety and agitation, in a manner similar to that described for the benzodiazepines. Hydroxyzine may be given orally or parenterally, while paraldehyde is preferably administered rectally.

In addition to the symptomatic control of the psychiatric manifestations of delirium, close attention must be paid to correcting any concomitant pathophysiological derangement, even though not directly related to the primary etiology of the delirium. The symptomatic treatment may involve a broad range of disturbances including fever, insomnia, cardiac arrhythmias, seizures, dehydration, nutritional deficits, and urinary retention.

Patient Management
The management of the delirious patient is the cornerstone of the total therapeutic approach. Its effectiveness is based on an understanding of the cognitive state of the patient and the factors that may influence it, as well as on an appreciation of the patient's psychological needs. Its goals are: (a) to optimize the patient's environment and the staff's bedside approach as a means of providing support to the patient's cognitive deficit, (b) to provide protection from accidents, and (c) to improve and maintain the patient's physical and mental state through nonspecific supportive measures that provide control and comfort. The key factor for successful management is the quality of nursing care.

In managing a delirious patient, one should be guided by the awareness that the patient is confused and disoriented; has impaired memory and cannot retain new information; has difficulty processing information; tends to misinterpret events and distort their meaning; cannot tolerate either excessive or diminished sensory input; and may be experiencing perceptual distortions in the form of illusions or even hallucinations that are often frightening.

The patient with a mild delirium of known etiology and good prognosis (e.g., idiosyncratic reaction to a drug, febrile illness) is best cared for at home, within a stable and familiar environment, and under the continuous care and supervision of family members. Patients with more serious deliria, and especially those of unknown etiology, require immediate hospitalization. The choice of hospital type depends on several considerations, including etiology of the underlying illness, degree and sophistication of medical and diagnostic requirements, and severity of behavioral disturbances. For instance, patients with a delirium due to serious physical illness (e.g., heart failure) should be treated in a general hospital; in the case of an alcohol withdrawal delirium, treatment may best be carried out in a detoxification unit; violent, suicidal, or acutely psychotic patients who show no evidence of serious physical illness require psychiatric hospitalization. Psychiatric consultation is required in most cases for assistance in diagnosis and management.

The *physical environment* should be stable and unambiguous, with elements that enhance familiarity and orientation, and maintain low sensory input, while at the same time preserving variability through stimulus change. The patient is best cared for in a quiet, simply furnished, and preferably single-bed room, softly lighted at all times, with mild stimulation provided by a radio or television set. A calendar, clock, and some personal articles (family pictures) should be at bedside for orientation and familiarity. Continuous supervision, preferably by a relative or friend who is thoroughly instructed about the requirements of this task, should be provided. Effort should be made to minimize the number of the nursing and house staff involved in the care of the patient, in order to increase the patient's familiarity with personnel. Special attention should be given to the overriding need for constant supervision and for instituting measures for protection from accidents, including suicidal and homicidal precautions when indicated. Physical restraints should be avoided whenever possible, and when applied they should be used for only brief periods. Control of agitation and combativeness is best managed by the personal contact of a supervising family member and by the appropriate use of tranquilizing drugs.

The interpersonal aspects of management are primarily determined by the patient's need to be oriented, to comprehend what is happening to him or her, and to be reassured. Accordingly, every interaction with the patient should adhere at all times to an approach that meets these needs. Professional staff should clearly identify themselves, state their role, remind the patient that he/she is in a hospital, and carefully explain what they intend to do. They should provide reassurance and explanation about everything that the patient experiences as alien, ambiguous, threatening, or frightening.

Upon recovery from the delirious state, the patient may have complete amnesia for the episode or may have spotty or incomplete recollection. If the patient is amnestic, he or she should be helped to understand the nature of the experiential gap and be reassured that his/her memory is now intact in spite of the amnesia. If the patient remembers the psychotic experiences (especially delusions and hallucinations), their nature and benign prognosis should be carefully explained.

SPECIFIC DISORDERS

292.81 Substance-induced Deliria

These are most common and are generally associated with substance abuse disorders, suicidal or accidental drug overdoses, and idiosyncratic reactions to drugs. The pathogenic mechanism depends on the pharmacologic action(s) of the drug. Predisposing or facilitating factors include age, biological substrate of the host, dosage, and route of administration. Clinically, they can be classified into three categories: (a) dose-related, (b) idiosyncratic, and (c) withdrawal deliria. This distinction allows definition of different approaches to treatment.

DOSE-RELATED DELIRIA

These are deliria induced by relatively high blood concentrations of a drug, secondary to acute overdose or repeated doses. Biological factors, such as age or capacity of the liver to metabolize drugs, contribute significantly as predisposing factors. The major treatment approach is the elimination of the causative agent from the body. Of major concern is the effect of the drug on various systems (cardiovascular, etc.) and counteracting these effects. DSM-III lists only two drug classes that cause delirium: amphetamine or similarly acting sympathomimetic drugs and phencyclidine (PCP) or similarly acting arylcyclohexylamines. There are, however, numerous other drugs that cause delirium, referred to in DSM-III as Other or Unspecified Substance Delirium (292.81).

Table 2 lists drugs that are known to cause delirium. Many of these drugs have anticholinergic action, the most common pharmacologic cause.

292.81 Amphetamine or Similarly Acting Sympathomimetic Delirium

This is part of the psychostimulant intoxication syndrome, developing within 24 hours of intake of stimulant drugs. Associated features include tactile and olfactory hallucinations, labile affect, and violent behavior. The delirium is short-lived, terminating in about six hours. Treatment and management are similar to that of intoxication by psychostimulant drugs (see Intoxications).

TABLE 2
Drugs Causing Delirium

Antidepressants (tricyclic, tetracyclic)—anticholinergic effect
    amitriptyline (Elavil, others)
    amoxapine (Asendin)
    desipramine (Pertofrane)
    doxepin (Sinequan, Adapin)
    imipramine (Tofranil, others)
    maprotiline (Ludiomil)
    nortriptyline (Aventyl)
    protriptyline (Vivactil)
    trimipramine (Surmontil)

Neuroleptics (low potency)—anticholinergic effect
    chlorpromazine (Thorazine, others)
    chlorprothixene (Taractan)
    mesoridazine (Serentil)
    thioridazine (Mellaril)

Antiparkinsonian—anticholinergic effect
    benztropine (Cogentin)
    trihexyphenidyl (Artane, others)
    biperiden HCL (Akineton)

Anticholinergics
    atropine
    belladonna alkaloids
    cyclopentolate (Cyclogyl)—eye drops
    scopolamine

Antihistamines—anticholinergic effect
    brompheniramine (Dimetane)
    diphenhydramine (Benadryl)
    hydroxyzine (Vistaril)
    over-the-counter sleep and cold medicines
    promethazine (Phenergan)

Anticonvulsants
    ethusuzimide (Zarontin)
    phenytoin (Dilantin, others)
    primidone (Mysoline)

TABLE 2 *(continued)*

Sympathomimetics
    amphetamines
    ephedrine
    phenylephrine
    methylphenidate (Ritalin)
    over-the-counter anorectics (phenetrazine, phenylpropanolamine,
      diethypropion)

Miscellaneous

aminocaproic acid (Amicar)	disulfiram (Antabuse)
amphotericin B (Fungizone)	ketamine (Ketalar)
asparaginase (Elspar)	levodopa (Dopar)
baclofen (Lioresal)	metrizamide (Amipaque)
chloroquine (Aralen)	phencyclidine (PCP)
cimetidine (Tagamet)	quinacrine (Atabrine)
corticosteroids (cortisone, pred- nisone, ACTH)	
cycloserine (Seromycin)	

**292.81 Phencyclidine (PCP) or Similarly Acting Arylcyclohexylamine
Delirium**
The delirium may develop within 24 hours after intake, or may emerge days
later after recovery from an overdose. It may last for a week with a waxing
and waning course. Associated features are those of phencyclidine intoxication. Treatment and management are described in the section on Intoxications.

Anticholinergic Substance Delirium
Drugs with anticholinergic activity include anticholinergics (atropine, sco-
polamine, etc.), antiparkinsonians (benztropine, trihexyphenidyl, etc.), tricyclic antidepressants (amitriptyline, imipramine, etc.), antihistamines, and
neuroleptics. Tricyclic drug overdose is a common cause of anticholinergic
delirium. Tricyclic plasma levels exceeding 300 ng/ml result in delirium in
50% of patients (Preskorn & Simpson, 1982). Treatment and management
are described in the section on Intoxications.

IDIOSYNCRATIC DELIRIA

These are not dose-related deliria. They occur early in the course of treatment at therapeutic doses. Genetically controlled enzymatic processes are thought to be responsible for the reaction (Balis, 1982). Many drugs may cause idiosyncratic deliria in predisposed individuals (see Table 2). They clear rapidly without any sequelae. Treatment is symptomatic.

WITHDRAWAL DELIRIA

This is a special class of substance-induced deliria involving a different pathogenic mechanism. They develop in individuals who have developed physiological dependence on alcohol, barbiturates, and other sedative-hypnotic drugs following prolonged use, and occur during withdrawal from the drug. Their treatment is discussed in the section on Withdrawal and Withdrawal Deliria.

293.00   Deliria Due to Other Etiologies

Most of the disorders listed in Table 1 may cause delirium. Metabolic disorders, systemic and CNS infections, head trauma, and postictal states are common etiologies. Their treatment is beyond the scope of this book.

DEMENTIAS

The term dementia, as currently used, does not carry the prognostic connotation of a progressive or irreversible course implied in the past. Depending on the underlying organic etiology, dementia may be reversible or irreversible. Its clinical course may be progressive, static, or remitting. Most of the causes of Organic Mental Disorders listed in Table 1 may produce dementia, either as a primary disorder (e.g., Primary Degenerative [Alzheimer's-type] Dementia) or as a secondary disorder, often progressing from an initial phase of delirium (e.g., protracted cerebral hypoxia, hypoglycemia).

The differentiation of reversible dementias, such as substance-induced disorders, deficiency disorders, benign intracranial masses, endocrine disorders, normal pressure hydrocephalus, epilepsy, CNS infections, Wilson's disease, Parkinson's disease, porphyria, chronic subdural hematoma, metabolic encephalopathies, or giant cerebral aneurysm is of great prognostic significance. Early diagnosis of these disorders is of utmost importance. Dementia must be differentiated from Delirium (no clouding of consciousness in dementia), Amnestic Syndrome (deficit involves only memory), and from the so-called "Pseudodementia," a form of depression masquerading as Dementia, which must always be ruled out before a diagnosis of dementia is made.

General Therapeutic Principles

The following general guidelines apply to the treatment and management of all dementias, with special emphasis on those arising in the senium. Treatment may be etiologic (when the cause is known and treatable) and/or symptomatic.

Etiologic Treatment

In searching for a treatable cause, first consideration should be given to ruling out depressive pseudodementia. A trial treatment with antidepressants may be justified in the absence of demonstrable etiology. The next step is to search for possible treatable organic causes (Cummings et al., 1980), especially when an etiologic diagnosis remains uncertain. This is particularly important in older patients, who are more likely to be diagnosed as suffering from Senile or Multi-infarct Dementia, often in the absence of any objective evidence. A diagnostic battery for screening etiologically treatable dementias often includes the following tests (McAllister & Price, 1982; Wells, 1979):

- Serology test for syphilis
- Complete blood count
- Serum B12, folate, T3 or T4
- Urinalysis
- Metabolic screen
- Drug screen
- Computerized axial tomography (CT-scan)

Additional examination and laboratory procedures may be needed.

Symptomatic Treatment

This is the only therapeutic approach available for those patients suffering from irreversible forms of dementia. Since the cognitive deficit of irreversible dementia is not amenable to any treatment, all therapeutic efforts are directed toward (a) improving impaired functions and promoting general health and (b) treating psychiatric complications, when they develop.

Demented patients, especially the elderly, must maintain the best possible physical health in order to prevent the consequences of physiological derangement on their already compromised cerebral functions. Every effort should be made to restore or improve impaired physical functions (e.g., renal, cardiovascular, respiratory, or endocrine), combat symptoms (pain, insomnia, constipation, impaired mobility), improve impaired hearing and vision, and maintain an optimal nutritional state. Of particular importance is the prevention of toxic effects of medication, prescribed or over-the-counter, and especially those resulting from drug interactions. Elderly patients are particularly susceptible to side effects because of decreased physiologic reserves and slower rates of absorption, metabolism and elimination of many drugs (Salzman et al., 1970). Demented patients are highly vulnerable to the development of secondary psychiatric disorders, including delirium, depression, and psychosis. The following is a brief review of the treatment of some common psychiatric problems in dementia.

Insomnia. This is a ubiquitous complaint of the elderly. Demented patients often cannot fall asleep as a result of becoming disoriented and frightened when the lights are turned out. The first measure to recommend is that of leaving a light on all night. Patients with sleep-onset insomnia may benefit from L-tryptophan, which can be prescribed as a pill or provided through high tryptophan foods such as milk, meat, or tuna fish. When drug treatment becomes necessary, antihistamines in low doses are the best tolerated (e.g., promethazine hydrochloride 25–50 mg or diphenhydramine 25–50 mg at bedtime) (Salzman, 1982). Thioridazine 25 mg is also effective and well tolerated. Chloral hydrate in doses 250–500 mg is recommended as the next least toxic drug. The hypnotic benzodiazepines (e.g., flurazepam), although the most widely prescribed hypnotics, work only for a few weeks, and some tend to produce unwanted daytime drowsiness, ataxia, confusion, and hallucinations at higher doses. Insomnia secondary to another disorder (e.g., depression) should be treated etiologically.

Anxiety, Irritability, Agitation. Irritability is common, especially in the early phase of senile dementia. Benzodiazepines are the drugs of choice for treating nonpsychotic anxiety states, when psychotherapeutic approaches fail to control the symptoms. In choosing a suitable benzodiazepine for the elderly demented patient, the clinician must take into consideration the kinetics and biotransformation of the various representatives of this class of anxiolytics (see Treatment section on Deliria). The long-acting chlordiazepoxide and diazepam are undesirable because of cumulative effects. The short-acting oxazepam and lorazepam are the preferred anxiolytic drugs, prescribed in approximately one-third to one-half of the younger adult dose. Excessive sedation, apathy, ataxia, incoordination, disorientation, confusion, and dysarthria are common toxic effects (Salzman, 1982).

Delirium. This is a most common psychiatric complication, especially in patients with Multi-infarct Dementia. Various drugs, especially anticholinergic, are very common causes of delirium in the elderly. For treatment, see section on Deliria.

Depression. Treatment of depression includes various psychotherapeutic approaches, antidepressant medication, and ECT (Ban, 1978b; Butler, 1975). In milder forms of dementia, supportive psychotherapy is useful in assisting the patient to grieve and accept cognitive losses and their consequences, and to maintain self-esteem. Psychotherapeutic management approaches are directed toward enhancing environmental-social support throughout the course of dementia. In the presence of severe depression, tri- or tetracyclic antidepressants are the preferred drugs. The choice of a specific tricyclic depends on clinical considerations as modified by the altered metabolism of the elderly. Several side effects of the tricyclics are especially hazardous for the elderly, because aging increases plasma half-life and steady-state plasma levels, especially with imipramine and amitriptyline (Robinson, 1979). Side effects include sedation, orthostatic hypotension, anticholinergic effects, and cardiotoxicity. The higher sedating effects of certain tricyclics (amitriptyline, doxepin) may be desirable in some patients for controlling insomnia, with the entire or two-thirds of the daily dose given before bedtime. The hypotensive effect of tricyclics does not seem to increase with advancing age (Glassman et al., 1979; Roose et al., 1981); nevertheless, orthostatic hypotension is a very common side effect and may precipitate falls, strokes, or heart attacks. Nortriptyline, compared with imipramine, produces less hypotension (Roose et al., 1981). Anticholinergic activity is especially prominent with amitriptyline, while desipramine, and to a lesser extent nortriptyline, have the least anticholinergic action. Elderly demented patients are particularly vulnerable to CNS anticholinergic toxicity, with one-third of patients on tricyclics being reported to develop confusion or delirium (Davies et al., 1971). Cardiotoxicity is of particular concern; tricyclics may produce sinus tachycardia, prolonged intraventricular conduction, and probably decreased myocardial contractility, as well as arrhythmias. Imipramine appears to have antiarrhythmic properties (Bigger et al., 1978).

In view of the above considerations, the tricyclics of choice are desipramine, nortriptyline, and doxepin, because they have the lowest relative toxicity. Of the three, desipramine is the least anticholinergic, and doxepin the least cardiotoxic (Salzman, 1982; Vohra et al., 1975). The so-called second-generation antidepressants (e.g., maprotiline, amoxapine, trazodone), which have been recently released for clinical use in this country, are reported to have fewer anticholinergic and cardiovascular side effects and therefore may present significant advantages over the older tricyclics in the treatment of the elderly patient (Gerner et al., 1980; Hrdina et al., 1980).

The following general guidelines apply in prescribing antidepressant drugs for the elderly demented patient:

1) Obtain pretreatment electrocardiogram and repeat ECG periodically during course of treatment.

2) Measure seated and standing blood pressure before treatment is started and before each increase in dose.

3) Start with very low doses (e.g., 30–40 mg, imipramine equivalent, daily in divided doses) and raise dose gradually, monitoring both therapeutic response and side effects (50–150 mg, imipramine equivalent, per day is the usual therapeutic range).

4) Give two-thirds of the dose before bedtime to promote sleep.

5) The concurrent administration of volume-depleting diuretics increases risk of exacerbation of orthostatic hypotension.

6) Exercise extreme caution in patients with preexisting cardiovascular disease and patients receiving quinidine or procainamide, and be fully familiar with contraindicated drug combinations (clonidine, guanethidine, or bethanidine).

7) Monitor tricyclic plasma levels regularly, in order to prevent cumulative toxic levels (Salzman, 1982).

Electroconvulsive therapy (ECT) may be indicated in depressed patients who fail to respond to an adequate course of treatment with antidepressants and patients who cannot tolerate the cardiotoxic effects of tricyclics (Salzman, 1975).

Psychosis. Psychotic symptoms are amenable to treatment with neuroleptic drugs, which, although equally effective in controlling psychotic thinking and behavior, differ in side effects and toxicity. As with the tricyclics, the choice of a specific antipsychotic agent should be based on considerations regarding toxicity and altered metabolism in the elderly (Salzman, 1982). Common side effects of neuroleptic drugs which may have serious consequences include sedation, orthostatic hypotension, anticholinergic effects, and extrapyramidal symptoms. Impaired thermoregulation and idiosyncratic reactions should also be noted.

Although the sedative effects of neuroleptics may be used therapeutically to induce sleep at night or tranquilize the agitated patient during daytime, they often produce confusion and disorientation in the elderly. Low potency neuroleptics (chlorpromazine, thioridazine, mesoridazine, chlorprothixene) have the strongest sedative effects, while the high potency neuroleptics (haloperidol, fluphenazine, perphenazine, trifluoperazine, and thiothixene) are least sedative. Low potency neuroleptics also have the strongest autonomic effects (hypotensive and anticholinergic) but show fewer extrapyramidal side effects. Conversely, high potency neuroleptics have minimal autonomic effects but very frequent extrapyramidal side effects. Although high potency neuroleptics (e.g., haloperidol) are generally safer and the drugs of choice in treating patients in whom autonomic and sedative effects are most hazardous, low potency neuroleptics (e.g., thioridazine) may be more appropriate for restless and agitated psychotic patients and those who are sensitive to extrapyramidal reactions. Elderly demented patients are particularly susceptible to the production of orthostatic hypotension (Blumenthal & Davie, 1980), as well as to central anticholinergic toxicity (confusion, delirium) and to extrapyramidal side effects (Hamilton, 1966; Salzman, 1982).

Neuroleptic treatment should begin with small amounts of the medication, given in divided doses (e.g., haloperidol 1–2 mg daily, or thioridazine 25–75 mg daily). In patients with violent or assaultive outbursts, propranolol may prove useful when other treatments have failed (Balis, 1979, 1982).

Patient Management
Effective management of the demented patient demands commitment on the part of the physician to accepting the responsibility for continuing care to a chronically ill and, in most instances, progressively deteriorating patient (Plutzky, 1974). The traditional medical model is expanded to include additional roles required for dealing with social and family problems confronting the patient and his/her caretakers. In this regard, the physician is often called upon to coordinate the activities of several caregivers including family members, social workers, visiting nurses, and other personnel in social service agencies. Knowledge of available community resources and how they can be utilized to benefit the total care of the demented patient is a prerequisite. Knowledge of the patient's medical and psychological needs, family resources and interpersonal dynamics, assets and liabilities, prognosis, and anticipated problems are all crucial for treatment planning.

The physician should maintain continuing interaction with family members, inform them about the patient's condition, advise them about proper management, and involve them in the patient's treatment. He or she should also provide them with emotional support and assist them in dealing with their feelings of shame, guilt, or anger, especially when they are called upon to make decisions for institutional placement of the patient. Relatives of the patient often become highly critical of the physician or nursing home staff as a means of coping with feelings of guilt or helplessness. These reaction patterns can be prevented or resolved through ventilation and moral support.

The doctor-patient relationship should remain a significant focus of the patient's management throughout the course of the illness. This is most important in the earlier phases of progressive dementias and in those patients with non-progressive dementias, such as those which follow an acute insult to the brain (e.g., head trauma, encephalitis, anoxia and hypoglycemic syndromes). The physician should structure each visit with the patient to provide psychological support by allaying fears, counteracting the sense of helplessness, allowing the ventilation of feelings, enhancing self-esteem, encouraging independence, strengthening healthier coping mechanisms, and correcting distortions of reality when present.

Rehabilitation through retraining is needed for those patients with milder residual deficit, in non-progressive dementias. Every effort should be made to maintain ambulation and prevent regression to wheelchair or bed. Other guidelines in the management of the demented patient include: encouragment of efforts toward a more independent and self-caring life-style, to the degree feasible; engagement in pleasurable, useful, or productive activities that enhance self-esteem; maintenance of preserved skills and abilities, as well as physical fitness; appropriate supervision to prevent consequences of cognitive impairment resulting from poor memory (e.g., fire hazards, getting lost, poor nutrition, deterioration of personal hygiene) or impaired social judgment (e.g., poor management of financial matters and personal affairs).

Appropriate manipulation of the patient's physical environment, whether in an institution or at home, is an important means of supporting impaired cognitive function, such as memory and orientation, and impaired sensory perception. Measures of environmental modulation to establish a "prosthetic environment" for the demented patient include good room lighting, with simple, stable, and familiar furnishings; clocks that sound the time and large calendars on the wall; note pads as memory aids; hearing aids; eyeglasses; dentures; hand rails; a walker, and so forth.

SPECIFIC DISORDERS

Irreversible Dementias
These are associated with permanent neuronal damage which may be (a) progressive or (b) residual (non-progressive).

(a) Progressive Dementias
These are irreversible dementias with a relentless course toward a vegetative state and death. They include Primary Degenerative Dementia, Senile and Presenile Onset (Alzheimer's type), Multi-infarct Dementia, and other less common disorders, such as Huntington's chorea, progressive supranuclear palsy, and so forth.

290.xx   Primary Degenerative Dementia, Senile Onset
290.1x   Primary Degenerative Dementia, Presenile Onset
This is the most common dementia affecting subjects of older age. Its etiology remains unknown. Some cases appear to have a familial occurrence. The dementia begins insidiously and progresses slowly, first with symptoms of memory loss, and later with symptoms of aphasia and apraxia, finally reaching a vegetative state after 8–10 years or longer. Compared to patients with Multi-infarct Dementia, patients with Alzheimer's Dementia seem to enjoy relatively good physical health.

Treatment is only symptomatic, as already described in the general section (Reisberg, 1982). A number of drugs have been reported as having a beneficial effect on the primary symptoms of cognitive deficit, although none of them has been proved to produce any significant or consistent effects. Acetylcholine deficit is of particular research interest as a possible mechanism of Primary Degenerative Dementias. So far, efforts to reverse or arrest cognitive deficit with the use of acetylcholine agonists or precursors have failed to provide significant results.

Studies involving the so-called nootropics, the choline precursor lecithin, piracetam, and ACTH-4-10 are currently underway (Cole & Braconnier, 1980; Reisberg et al., 1981; Salzman, 1979). Numerous other drugs have been used in the treatment of senile and presenile dementias with questionable results, including central nervous system stimulants (e.g., pentylenetetrazol, amphetamines, and amphetamine-like drugs), vasodilators (e.g., papaverine), anabolic substances, Hydergine, and other drugs (Ban, 1978a; Lehman & Ban, 1975; Yesavage, 1979). The use of the dihydrogenated ergot alkaloid, dihydroergotoxine mesylate (Hydergine), in sublingual doses of 1–2 mg three times daily, has recently received some support as a means of improving cognitive function in the early phase of senile dementia. Another popular drug is pentylenetetrazol given orally in doses of 200 mg three or four times daily. Proper patient management and family counseling are essential, and the only substantive services the physician can offer (Reisberg et al., 1981).

290.4x   Multi-infarct Dementia
This is the second most common of the progressive dementias arising in the senium. It is thought to be due to widespread multiple cerebral infarctions, secondary to cerebral arteriosclerosis. Hypertension is a very common concomitant disorder. There is no known effective method for reversing or arresting the course of this dementia. Various drugs, such as anticoagulants, vasodilators (Hydergine, papaverine), and lipotropic enzymes have been proposed for altering the course of vascular disease (Cole & Braconnier, 1980; Lehman & Ban, 1975; Salzman, 1982). No controlled studies have been

reported that clearly prove the value of any of these agents. Recent reports on the potential usefulness of antiplatelet-agglutinating drugs, such as acetylsalicylic acid (aspirin), in reducing the risk of infarction in patients with transient ischemic attacks may have some relevance in the treatment of Multi-infarct Dementia (Cole & Braconnier, 1980; Gaitz et al., 1977).

(b) Residual Non-Progressive Dementias

These include dementias that develop after an acute brain insult. Etiologic and symptomatic treatment should aim at preventing further brain damage during the acute phase. One should allow sufficient time for partial reversal of neuronal injury before any deficit is declared permanent.

Reversible (Treatable) Dementias

These dementias are of great clinical significance because the underlying cerebral disorder can be arrested or fully reversed if appropriate etiologic treatment is applied (Cummings et al., 1980). Eminently treatable are the substance-induced dementias (e.g., chronic intoxication with bromides or barbiturates, etc.) and dementias due to metabolic encephalopathies, hypothyroidism, chronic subdural hematoma, congestive heart failure, meningiomas, vitamin deficiency (e.g., pernicious anemia), hypertensive encephalopathy, carotid artery occlusal disease, and so forth. Other treatable dementias include those associated with normal pressure hydrocephalus, Parkinson's disease, Wilson's disease, and epilepsy. Discussion of the specific etiologic treatment of each of these disorders is beyond the scope of this book.

AMNESTIC SYNDROMES

The amnestic syndrome is an Organic Brain Syndrome characterized by a selective cognitive impairment in short- and long-term memory. The syndrome occurs in a state of clear awareness (differentiating it from Delirium) and without any significant loss of the remaining intellectual abilities (differentiating it from Dementia).

The syndrome results from bilateral lesions of specific diencephalic or medial temporal lobe structures (e.g., hippocampal formation, mammillary bodies, fornix, and structures in the floor and walls of the third ventricle). The lesions may be reversible or irreversible, depending on the etiology of the causative disorder. Conditions associated with Amnestic Syndrome of either transient or persistent course include thiamine deficiency (e.g., Wernicke-Korsakoff syndrome), head trauma, carbon monoxide poisoning, subarachnoid hemorrhage, herpes simplex encephalitis, brain tumors, bilateral posterior cerebral arterial occlusion, cerebral hypoxia, and surgical excision. Conditions associated with transient amnestic syndrome include temporal lobe epilepsy, migraine attacks, chronic drug intoxication (e.g., barbiturates, bromides, isoniazid), and electroconvulsive therapy.

General Therapeutic Principles

The following guidelines apply to the treatment and management of Amnestic Syndrome. Treatment is etiologic (when cause is known and treatable) and symptomatic.

Etiologic Treatment

This involves the identification and specific treatment of the underlying primary disorder. In some instances, preventive treatment is of major importance (e.g., epilepsy, alcoholism, drug abuse, migraine).

Symptomatic Treatment

There is no symptomatic treatment to correct the cognitive deficit in memory. Physostigmine may improve the Amnestic Syndrome after herpes simplex encephalitis (Peters & Levin, 1977). Memory therapy (teaching the patient to use visual mnemonics) may be helpful to patients with preserved ability to retrieve visual images (Patten, 1972).

Patient Management

Management approaches are similar to those described for demented patients. However, it should be noted that, compared with demented patients, amnestic patients suffer from a more circumscribed cognitive deficit, maintain relatively intact verbal capacities, and are less vulnerable to developing major psychiatric complications. Although institutionalized custodial care may be necessary for patients with more severe forms, most of these patients can be cared for at home or in a supervised, structured environment. Efforts at rehabilitation of patients with milder syndromes should always be part of the management plan.

SPECIFIC DISORDERS

Transient Amnestic Syndromes

The substance-induced amnestic syndromes and those due to epilepsy, migraine, and mild head trauma are eminently treatable using the procedures outlined above.

(a) **Substance-Induced.** The most commonly implicated drugs are seda-tive-hypnotics. Other drugs include isoniazid, bromides, and arsenic.

**292.83   Barbiturate or Similarly Acting Sedative or Hypnotic
Amnestic Disorder**
Discontinuation of the drug leads to full recovery (see Intoxications). Treat-ment of drug abuse and rehabilitation are indispensable aspects of manage-ment (see Substance Use Disorders).

(b) **Other Transient Amnestic Syndromes.**

Temporal Lobe Epilepsy Amnestic Syndrome
This is characterized by brief amnestic episodes that rarely persist for hours and during which the EEG shows ictal dysrhythmia attributed to seizure foci localized in the limbic system. Treatment aims at effective control with ap-propriate anticonvulsant drugs.

Relatively Irreversible Amnestic Syndromes
The irreversibility of an amnestic syndrome depends on the severity of the acute insult to the brain, the duration of the noxious effect, and the delay in instituting specific treatment. Such conditions include head trauma with damage to diencephalic or temporal regions; brain tumors encroaching on the same cerebral regions; bilateral hippocampal infarctions due to thrombo-sis or embolism of posterior cerebral arteries; herpes simplex encephalitis; and cerebral anoxic states. Review of the treatment of these disorders is be-yond the scope of the book.

The most common form of amnestic syndrome is that associated with thiamine deficiency secondary to prolonged, heavy use of alcohol. Thiamine deficiency may also be observed in individuals with poor nutritional status, such as the neglected elderly and those on vitamin-deficient diets.

291.10   Alcohol Amnestic Disorder
This thiamine deficiency syndrome, also known as Korsakoff's Disease, is secondary to the nutritional deficit associated with chronic alcoholism. In the majority of cases, the onset is acute, presenting as a sequela of Wernicke's en-cephalopathy; a small number of patients show an insidious onset without a preceding acute encephalopathic episode.

The reversibility of the Wernicke-Korsakoff syndrome depends on the promptness of instituting specific treatment with thiamine. Thiamine should initially be given parenterally in doses of 50 mg daily for about one week and then be switched to an oral administration, provided the patient is able to resume a normal diet. This treatment should be continued for several months, together with a supplement of B-complex vitamins. Follow-up studies report that about one-fourth of Wernicke-Korsakoff cases recover completely, one-fourth fail to show any improvement, and half of the cases have partial recovery with varying degrees of residual memory deficit (Victor et al., 1971).

ORGANIC HALLUCINOSES
Organic hallucinosis is a syndrome characterized by recurrent or persistent hallucinations attributable to a specific organic factor judged to be etiologically related to the disturbance. The hallucinations are the only essential feature, occurring in a state of clear awareness (differentiating it from delirium) and in the absence of a formal thought disturbance.

Specific conditions producing organic hallucinosis include substance abuse (e.g., alcohol, hallucinogens, cocaine), drug toxicity (e.g., levodopa, bromocriptine), temporal lobe epilepsy, space-occupying lesions of the brain, migraine, temporal arteritis, loss of hearing or vision, and other situations involving sensory deprivation. The course and prognosis of organic hallucinosis vary greatly, depending on the underlying pathology.

General Therapeutic Principles
The treatment and management of patients with organic hallucinosis are similar to those of other Organic Mental Disorders.

Treatment
The major focus is on identification of the underlying specific disorder in order to be able to institute appropriate etiologic treatment. The most common etiology is substance abuse, especially alcohol and hallucinogens, but other sources must of course be sought.

Methods of symptomatic control of hallucinations vary according to the underlying source of the disturbance. For instance, ictal hallucinations and hallucinogen flashbacks may be controlled with antiepileptic drugs. A patient suffering from alcoholic hallucinosis may require treatment with neuroleptics. Neuroleptics are also recommended for the control of paranoid delusions that may accompany the hallucinosis. Reactive psychopathology may require psychotherapy, generally of a supportive nature.

Patient Management
Management approaches must be directed toward both the underlying illness and the reactive psychopathology which may be present. Patients with substance abuse require special efforts to engage them in a comprehensive reha-

bilitation program (see Substance Use Disorders). Epileptics have special psychological, social, and vocational needs that should be dealt with as part of their total treatment plan. Patients suffering from irreversible loss of vision or hearing may require appropriate social stimulation to counteract the partial sensory deprivation.

Reactive psychopathology may require psychiatric management. Anxious, agitated, or frightened patients must be calmed down and reassured that their symptoms are transient. Suicidal tendencies or extreme fear or agitation may make hospitalization necessary.

SPECIFIC DISORDERS

Substance-induced Hallucinosis
The most commonly implicated substances are alcohol and hallucinogens.

291.30   Alcohol Hallucinosis
Alcoholic Hallucinosis consists of vivid auditory hallucinations developing shortly (usually within 48 hours) after cessation or reduction of heavy ingestion of alcohol in an individual who apparently has alcohol dependence. The course usually consists of an acute phase lasting in typical cases less than one week, but in some cases (25%) it may be followed by a chronic phase that may last several months, even years, and may be clinically indistinguishable from schizophrenia. In previous definitions, the acute form was thought to be part of the withdrawal syndrome, while the chronic form was diagnosed as schizophrenia.

Treatment of the acute phase is similar to that of alcohol withdrawal (see Treatment section on Withdrawal and Withdrawal Deliria). The "detoxification" procedure includes control of anxiety and agitation, rest, vitamins, and nutritional supplements. The chronic form is treated with neuroleptic drugs and supportive psychotherapy in a manner similar to that of Schizophreniform Disorder.

305.30   Hallucinogen Hallucinosis
This refers to the typical "trip" induced by hallucinogen intoxication (LSD, MDT, mescaline, psilocybin, etc.). Large doses of cannabis or tetrahydrocannabinol (THC) may also result in hallucinosis. The duration of the syndrome varies according to the type of hallucinogen, lasting about six hours for LSD, and from under an hour to a day or two for other hallucinogens. If the syndrome persists longer than 24 hours, it is classified as a Hallucinogen

Delusional Disorder or a Hallucinogen Affective Disorder, depending on whether the symptoms are delusional or affective in nature (see corresponding sections below).

The treatment and management of Hallucinogen Hallucinosis are the same as for the "bad tripper" (Berger & Tinklenberg, 1979; Greenblatt & Shader, 1975; Solursh & Clement, 1968; Taylor et al., 1975). These patients are typically seen in emergency rooms, frequently brought in by friends or the police. The physician should be familiar with the street patterns of drug abuse, the current code names of various illicit drugs, and their clinical manifestations. The first step is to place the patient in a quiet room under supervision. The patient needs protection from external stimulation and from the potential consequences of his or her maladaptive behavior. The second step is to attempt to identify the nature of the drug taken, the amount involved, and the time that has elapsed since it was ingested. It is also helpful to inquire about previous exposures to hallucinogens and the patient's reaction to them. Information obtained from either the patient or friends is very often unreliable because of possible legal implications and inability to define the actual drug agent and its purity. Illicit drugs are frequently adulterated ("cut") with other toxic drugs, such as atropine and strychnine, a fact that may present serious treatment complications, especially if the patient is treated with anticholinergic drugs.

The symptom that usually brings the patient to the emergency room is the fear that he or she is going to "lose control" or that he or she will "never come down." This frightening feeling is further aggravated by bizarre illusions and hallucinations, depersonalization, distortions of the body image, and delusions. There are two types of treatment approaches in managing the "bad tripper": (a) the "talk-down" method, and (b) the use of medications. Generally, the "talk-down" method is the recommended one, because medications may aggravate a state of intoxication of obscure etiology.

(a) **Talk-down Method.** The basic goal is to provide continuing reassurance and reality-defining through the establishment of verbal contact with the patient. The therapist tries to reassure the patient about the transient nature of the experience and the forthcoming "coming down"; provides empathic support; and repetitively defines the reality of the patient's experience, reducing distortions, while the patient is encouraged to describe what is happening to him or her. Communications should consist of repeated, simple, concrete statements. As the patient is improving, he/she should be told to anticipate an "in-and-out" phase during which there is a waxing and waning of awareness. This method requires considerable time and effort that may not be available in an emergency room situation (Berger & Tinklenberg, 1979; Greenblatt & Shader, 1975; Taylor et al., 1975).

(b) **Use of Medications.** The use of drugs is recommended when the patient is inaccessible or fails to respond to verbal contact, or when there is not sufficient time to spare for "talking him down." Neuroleptics are contraindicated, although effective, primarily because of their anticholinergic effects which are likely to precipitate an anticholinergic crisis in the event that the illicit drug was adulterated with atropine or other anticholinergic substances (Gershon et al., 1965). Benzodiazepines are the drugs of choice (e.g., diazepam in doses of 20–30 mg orally, repeated every three to six hours as necessary for controlling anxiety and agitation) (Berger & Tinklenberg, 1979; Taylor et al., 1975). Short-acting barbiturates are also effective, but should be avoided because of risk of respiratory depression. Upon recovery from the acute episode, the patient should be discharged to the custody and care of a responsible person with the advice to stay home for 24 hours. He/she should also be offered the opportunity for referral to a drug treatment program. Overnight hospitalization may be advisable for the patient who fails to respond to the above treatment approaches and continues to show perceptual and cognitive disturbances. Continuation of these symptoms beyond 24 hours requires a revision of the initial diagnosis (e.g., to Organic Delusional Syndrome).

Hallucinogen-induced intermittent hallucinoses (flashbacks) are spontaneous episodic recurrences of perceptual, cognitive, or affective disturbances which were originally experienced during acute hallucinogen intoxication. The phenomenon is thought to be due to a kindling effect of specific internal or external stimuli on temporolimbic structures whose seizure threshold was lowered by repeated effects of hallucinogens. Benzodiazepines in low doses have been reported to be effective in controlling flashbacks (Berger & Tinklenberg, 1979). Similarly, anticonvulsant drugs (e.g., phenytoin) have also been found effective (Ifabumuyi & Jeffries, 1976).

Chronic hallucinatory psychosis is refractory to neuroleptic treatment; it has been reported, however, to respond to anticonvulsant drugs (Ifabumuyi & Jeffries, 1976). Treatment with benzodiazepines may also be justified if anticonvulsants prove ineffective after adequate trial.

292.12   Other Substance-induced Hallucinosis

Most of the drugs listed in Table 2 may produce organic hallucinosis. Those most commonly implicated include amantadine, baclofen, bromocriptine, ephedrine, propranolol, pentazocine, and levodopa. The syndrome is generally benign and transient, rapidly subsiding after discontinuation of the drug.

Mild sedation with a benzodiazepine drug may become necessary for the anxious and agitated patient (see Deliria).

293.82 Miscellaneous Conditions Producing Hallucinosis

Temporal lobe epilepsy, migraine, temporal arteritis, space-occupying lesions of the brain, and posterior cerebral artery occlusion (Brust, 1977) may be associated with hallucinosis (Lipowski, 1980a). Of particular diagnostic interest are those patients who experience only hallucinatory auras without a history of psychomotor seizures. Treatment of ictal hallucinosis should be directed toward the primary lesion (e.g., if amenable to surgery) and the control of seizural episodes with anticonvulsants. The reader is referred elsewhere for the treatment of other conditions (Brust, 1977).

Patients with partial sensory deprivation (loss of vision or hearing) may also experience "release-type" hallucinations. Treatment should be aimed at correcting the primary disorder (e.g., surgery for cataract, hearing aids). If the disorder is not amenable to treatment, an effort should be made to enrich the patient's environment through appropriate social stimulation.

ORGANIC DELUSIONAL SYNDROMES

The Organic Delusional Syndrome is characterized by delusions that are judged to be due to a specific organic factor. Diagnosis of the syndrome involves presumption rather than definitive diagnosis; the "organic" nature of some of these disorders remains controversial. Course and prognosis depend on the underlying pathology.

General Therapeutic Principles

The treatment of patients with Organic Delusional Syndrome is both etiologic and symptomatic, while their management is similar to that of functional psychoses.

Treatment

As with other Organic Mental Disorders, the primary focus is on the diagnosis of a specific causative factor presumed to be responsible for the syndrome. The most common etiology is amphetamine abuse. Other common disorders that should be considered early include epilepsy, pernicious anemia, hypo- or hyperthyroidism, systemic lupus erythematosus, neurosyphilis, and brain tumors. Most of these are amenable to specific treatment.

Symptomatic treatment should control delusions and agitation, as well as the physical symptoms of the underlying pathology (e.g., control of seizures in epilepsy).

In general, effective control of the delusions and other psychotic symptoms may be achieved with neuroleptic drugs (see general guidelines applicable to schizophrenic and paranoid disorders). In some disorders, symptomatic treatment of psychosis may involve drugs of greater specificity, such as anticonvulsants in epilepsy and propranolol in porphyria (Atsmon & Blum, 1978). Supportive psychotherapy and other psychosocial approaches follow the same general guidelines applicable to the treatment of functional psychoses.

Patient Management
The management of patients with Organic Delusional Syndrome is similar to that of patients with schizophrenic, schizophreniform, and paranoid disorders.

SPECIFIC DISORDERS
The following is a brief review of the most commonly encountered organic delusional syndromes of specific etiology.

Substance-induced Delusional Disorders

292.11   Amphetamine or Similarly Acting Sympathomimetic Delusional Disorder
The treatment of the acute phase is primarily supportive, unless the patient is agitated, in which case neuroleptics may be used. Persistent delusions and flashbacks are treated with neuroleptics. Some patients may later experience recurrent flashbacks of delusional ideas, often triggered by small doses of amphetamines.

292.11   Hallucinogen Delusional Disorder
Symptomatic treatment of the Hallucinogen Delusional Disorder follows the guidelines applicable to schizophrenic and paranoid disorders (see also Hallucinogen Hallucinosis).

292.11   Cannabis Delusional Disorder
Treatment is similar to that of the "bad tripper" (see Hallucinogen Hallucinosis).

292.90   Phencyclidine (PCP) or Similarly Acting Arylcyclohexylamine Mixed Organic Mental Disorder
Although a mixed syndrome involving features of several Organic Brain Syndromes, it is described here because it often evolves into an Organic Delusional Syndrome. The Delusional Syndrome closely resembles chronic schizo-

phrenia. Patients with PCP psychosis often require physical restraints during the intoxication or delirious state, because of the risk of violent or suicidal behavior.

The treatment of PCP psychosis involves overcoming psychiatric manifestations and clearing PCP from the body. There is evidence that PCP is stored in lipids of the brain and other organs where it may be retained up to a year after the last known contact (Aniline et al., 1981). Urinary acidifiers such as ammonium chloride are effective in clearing PCP from the blood. However, acidification for several weeks until no PCP is detectable in the urine or blood does not rid the lipids of stored PCP. Periodic forced urine acidification may be required in an effort to clear the lipid stores of PCP, especially in those patients who experience flashbacks. These recrudescences of symptoms occur with febrile illnesses, exercise, emotional distress, or the ingestion of certain foods and are thought to result from reintoxication from mobilized PCP in lipid stores. Urine acidification (pH below 5) can be accomplished by the administration of ammonium chloride in doses of 500 mg three or four times daily until PCP disappears from the urine and blood (Berger & Tinklenberg, 1979; Lewis & Senay, 1981).

Diazepam is the drug of choice for symptomatic treatment of psychotic manifestations. During the acute phase, 10–30 mg of diazepam orally or intramuscularly may be required to control violent behavior. Smaller doses given daily in divided doses are indicated in the persistent forms. Neuroleptics are also effective in controlling psychotic symptoms; however, the low potency neuroleptics (e.g., chlorpromazine, thioridazine) should be avoided because of the risk of potentiating the anticholinergic effects of PCP. Haloperidol is the preferred neuroleptic for the control of both psychotic and assaultive behavior. The rapid neuroleptization method discussed elsewhere in this book may be applied during the acute phase (Berger & Tinklenberg, 1979; Lewis & Senay, 1981). (See also PCP Delirium and Intoxication).

292.11   Other or Unspecified Substance-induced Delusional Disorder

Numerous prescribed drugs may induce an Organic Delusional Syndrome as a result of excessive dosage or idiosyncratic intoxication. The most common include asparaginase, bromocriptine, bromides, chloroquine, cimetidine, corticosteroids, cycloserine, digitalis glycosides, disopyramide, disulfiram, indomethacin, isoniazid, levodopa, methyldopa, pentazocine, phenelzine, propranolol, and sulindac (*The Medical Letter*, 1981). With the exception of bromide psychosis, the psychotic reaction is transient, requiring only brief symptomatic treatment (e.g., haloperidol), following discontinuation of the implicated drug or reduction of the dosage in the event that its continuous use is mandatory.

Miscellaneous Organic Delusional Syndromes

Non-substance-induced Organic Delusional Syndromes (293.81) include temporal lobe epilepsy, pernicious anemia, brain tumors, hypo- or hyperthyroidism, hypoparathyroidism, Cushing's syndrome, systemic lupus erythematosus, prophyria, head trauma, Huntington's chorea, and CNS infections (encephalitis, neurosyphilis) (Lipowski, 1975, 1980a).

Epileptic psychosis is a complication of temporal lobe epilepsy, developing in a small percentage of patients many years after the onset of seizures (Balis, 1978; Blumer, 1975, 1977). Psychotic and seizural episodes may show an inverse relationship in a seesaw phenomenon. During the psychotic episode the EEG shows "forced normalization." Neuroleptic drugs are of little usefulness, with some notable rare exceptions. Reduction of the dosage of anticonvulsant drugs as a means of allowing the occurrence of seizures may be advisable in those patients whose psychosis is inversely related to seizure frequency. Induction of a grand mal seizure by ECT has been suggested.

It is beyond the scope of this book to review the treatment of other specific conditions.

ORGANIC AFFECTIVE SYNDROMES

The diagnosis of Organic Affective Syndrome also involves a presumptive rather than definitive diagnosis. Etiologic factors include various drugs (e.g., reserpine, corticosteroids), endocrine diseases (e.g., Cushing's syndrome), pernicious anemia, hypothyroidism, infectious diseases (e.g., influenza), brain tumors, Parkinson's disease, carcinoma of the pancreas, temporal lobe epilepsy, and other conditions. It should be noted that these factors may also produce other Organic Brain Syndromes. Course and prognosis depend on the underlying pathology.

General Therapeutic Principles

Treatment is both etiologic and symptomatic, as is the case with all Organic Brain Syndromes.

Treatment

Etiologic treatment of the underlying pathology does not promptly reverse the affective syndrome. The latter may persist for weeks or months after successful recovery from the primary disease.

Symptomatic treatment is directed toward the removal of the symptoms of the affective syndrome (depression, mania), as well as the physical symptoms of the primary disorder. The treatment of the affective syndrome follows the general guidelines applicable to the functional affective disorders. Psychopharmacological treatment often involves the use of tri- or tetracyclic antidepressants. ECT may be advisable in cases refractory to drugs, when suicidal risk is imminent, or when antidepressant drug toxicity is hazardous or intolerable, as in the case of serious cardiac disease. In some disorders, such as temporal lobe epilepsy, the control of the depressive episode may involve drugs of greater specificity (e.g., anticonvulsants). Supportive psychotherapy and other psychosocial approaches follow the same guidelines applicable to the treatment of functional depressive disorders.

Lithium carbonate has been reported to be effective in various organic manic syndromes including those associated with steroids and other drugs (Falk et al., 1979), Cushing's syndrome, and metabolic disturbances (Krauthammer & Klerman, 1978). Neuroleptics (e.g., haloperidol) may also be effective and should be tried in patients unresponsive to lithium. Carbamazepine has been recently reported to be very effective in the treatment of bipolar patients. A trial of carbamazepine is justified when the patient fails to respond to lithium or when lithium toxicity is intolerable. It should be the drug of choice for ictal manic episodes in patients with temporal lobe epilepsy (Troupin, 1978).

Patient Management
The management of patients with Organic Affective Syndrome is similar to that of patients with functional affective disorders. Suicide risk in the depressed patient and socially disruptive behavior in the manic may necessitate psychiatric hospitalization.

SPECIFIC DISORDERS
Organic Affective Disorders may be divided into substance-induced and those of other etiology.

Substance-induced Affective Disorder

292.84 Hallucinogen Affective Disorder
Treatment follows the general guidelines applicable to affective disorders.

292.84 Other or Unspecified Substance-induced Affective Disorder
The most commonly implicated are antihypertensive drugs, steroids, amphetamines, and phencyclidine. Other sources are too numerous to address specifically here. General guidelines may be inferred from the text above.

Antihypertensive Drugs. Reserpine, methyldopa, guanethidine, clonidine, bethanidine, and alpha-blockers (propranolol) have been reported to cause depression (Whitlock & Evans, 1978). Reserpine is the most commonly implicated, precipitating a major depressive episode in 5% of patients treated. Treatment involves discontinuation of the drug and the use of antidepressants or ECT if the depression does not remit promptly.

Steroid Drugs. Corticosteroids, ACTH, and oral contraceptives have been reported to cause affective syndromes. Reduction of dosage may result in improvement; in the event that the drug cannot be discontinued, mania can be effectively controlled with lithium treatment. Lithium may also provide prophylaxis against steroid-induced affective syndrome (Falk et al., 1979). Neuroleptics (e.g., perphenazine, haloperidol) have also been used as effective means of controlling mania. The treatment of depression with tricyclics may produce delirium in such patients; it is advisable to use small doses and monitor the plasma levels of the drug regularly.

Other. Depressive syndromes following amphetamine withdrawal and in PCP psychosis are discussed elsewhere.

293.83   Other Organic Affective Disorders
Other conditions associated with Organic Affective Syndrome include endocrine diseases (Gold et al., 1981), temporal lobe epilepsy, systemic lupus erythematosus, brain tumors, pernicious anemia, Parkinson's disease, Huntington's chorea, carcinoid syndrome, carcinoma of the pancreas, and postviral syndromes (influenza, infectious mononucleosis, infectious hepatitis, viral pneumonia) (Lipowski, 1980a, b). Symptomatic treatment of the affective syndrome in these disorders should follow the guidelines above.

ORGANIC PERSONALITY SYNDROMES
The Organic Personality Syndrome is characterized by marked change in personality and behavior that is judged to be due to a specific organic factor antedating the onset of the syndrome. The cardinal feature is disinhibition with impaired control of the expression of emotions and impulses. The most common causes are head trauma, cerebrovascular disease, and space-occupying lesions of the brain. Other causes include temporal lobe epilepsy, multiple sclerosis, chronic intoxications (e.g., cannabis, LSD, steroids), endocrine disorders (e.g., hypercalcemia), chronic poisoning (e.g., mercury, manganese), neurosyphilis, post-encephalitic parkinsonism, and Huntington's chorea. The course and prognosis depend on the underlying pathology (Lipowski, 1980a, b).

General Therapeutic Principles

Treatment is etiologic (if the underlying condition is treatable) and sympto-matic. Management approaches should aim at enhancing behavioral control and minimizing undesirable conduct.

Treatment

Etiologically treatable conditions include endocrine diseases, substance-in-duced disorders, space-occupying lesions of the brain, epilepsy, and neuro-syphilis.

Symptomatic treatment should control emotional lability and impulse dyscontrol, as well as the physical symptoms of the underlying disorder.

Explosive outbursts of anger and episodes of violent behavior that occur with minimal provocation are the most serious symptoms. Pharmacologic control of these may be possible with the use of lithium, propranolol, anti-convulsant drugs, carbamazepine, or neuroleptics (Balis, 1979; Kuhn, 1976; Puente, 1976). Lithium has been reported to have a nonspecific therapeutic effect on aggressive and violent behavior (Marini & Sheard, 1977; Sheard, 1975; Sheard et al., 1976; Tupin, 1978). Propranolol may control violent epi-sodes in patients with closed-head brain injury and those with temporal lobe epilepsy. Anticonvulsant drugs (Monroe, 1975), and especially carbamaze-pine (alone or in combination with propranolol), have been shown to im-prove irritability and episodic rage in patients with temporolimbic epilepsy (Kuhn, 1976; Troupin, 1978; Tunks & Dermer, 1977). Neuroleptic drugs, al-though used extensively, are usually ineffective.

Psychosocial therapeutic approaches, including individual psychother-apy, group and family therapy, and behavior modification techniques, have been reported to be of value in the treatment of some of these patients.

Patient Management

The management of the patient with Organic Personality Syndrome is pri-marily directed towards enhancing behavioral controls and minimizing un-desirable conduct at work or within family and social settings. This may be accomplished through direct counseling and family intervention.

Patient counseling should help the patient avoid situations that trigger violent outbursts; abstain from alcohol, which may induce dyscontrol epi-sodes; learn ways to prevent social embarrassment; and make decisions about job changes or early retirement, if necessary. Vocational rehabilitation may be indicated.

Family counseling is an essential part of management. Family members need to be advised about the changes in the patient's personality, especially with regard to behavioral dyscontrol and impaired social judgment (e.g., the likelihood of embarrassing behaviors, shoplifting, sexual indiscretions, or sexual abuse of minors). The physician should provide emotional support for their caring for the needs of the patient, as well as for their own needs (Lezak, 1978). The physician should advise about proper management of the patient and assist in developing coping strategies and/or in avoiding situations that tend to elicit psychopathology. It is most important that the family understand the interaction of environmental contingencies (e.g., supports and demands of social situations) with the patient's life-long pattern of coping style in the face of organic disinhibition (Leigh, 1979). For instance, excessive obsessiveness and "viscosity" in the epileptic personality may represent compensatory mechanisms for maintaining control in the face of uncontrollable seizures; occurrence of "catastrophic reactions" (crying, rage, or cognitive disorganization) may be manifest when the brain-injured person is faced with the charge of performing tasks beyond his or her capabilities. The patient should be allowed to perform at his or her level of capability, in his or her own tedious and ruminative style, and in a familiar setting that provides routine and predictability. Novelty and excessive stimulus change in a shifting environment strain the patient's capabilities, and the ensuing stress often leads to reactive psychopathology. Patients who are violent, sexually abusive to minors, or otherwise unmanageable may have to be removed from the home.

SPECIFIC DISORDERS
The DSM-III lists two syndromatic categories (substance-induced and other) without any reference to specific disorders.

292.89   Other or Unspecified Substance Personality Disorder
Therapeutic approaches for patients with substance abuse should involve a comprehensive drug rehabilitation program with efforts toward social and vocational rehabilitation and resocialization (see Substance Use Disorders). In other cases, the guidelines already described should be followed.

310.10   Other Organic Personality Syndrome

Head Trauma. In the milder forms of a post-concussion syndrome, emotional lability (e.g., uncontrollable crying, angry outbursts, irritability) may be controlled with propranolol or psychostimulants (e.g., methylphenidate). Treatment and management of more severe syndromes were briefly discussed in the preceding section on General Therapeutic Principles.

Temporal Lobe Epilepsy. Anticonvulsant drugs (e.g., carbamazepine) may improve hypersexuality and irritability (Troupin, 1978). Propranolol (alone or in combination with carbamazepine) may be effective in controlling rage outbursts (Balis, 1979; Kuhn, 1976; Tunks & Dermer, 1977). Psychotherapy and family counseling are of value for some patients (Blumer, 1977).

Other Causes. *Chronic hypercalcemia* due to hyperparathyroidism or other causes may be fully reversed with correction of the hypercalcemia (Peterson, 1968). Cerebral neoplasms (e.g., meningiomas pressing on the frontal lobes), subarachnoid hemorrhage, especially with anterior communicating artery aneurysm (Storey, 1970), neurosyphilis, and Wilson's disease are other examples of treatable disorders.

WITHDRAWAL AND WITHDRAWAL DELIRIA
Withdrawal includes all manifestations of the "abstinence sickness" except delirium. The syndrome varies according to the substance involved. Common symptoms include anxiety, restlessness, irritability, insomnia, and impaired attention. The nature of the substance determines additional symptoms which are characteristic of that particular substance or of its class. The course of withdrawal is generally self-limited, unless it becomes complicated by Delirium. *Withdrawal Delirium* is a complication of certain substance-specific withdrawal syndromes associated with dependence on alcohol or hypnotic-sedative drugs. Withdrawal from alcohol or hypnotic-sedative drugs may be complicated by delirium and grand mal seizures.

General Therapeutic Principles
The ultimate goal of the treatment is to eliminate the state of physiological dependence without allowing the occurrence of the withdrawal syndrome. The procedure by which this is accomplished is called *detoxification.* This procedure is based on the principle of gradually withdrawing an individual from the drug by means of administering decreasing doses, either of the same drug on which the individual is dependent or one that is cross-tolerant to it (Czechowicz, 1978). Loss of substance dependence does not necessarily cure the underlying Substance Use Disorder. The most important factor of substance abuse is the mechanism of psychological dependence, in which complex underlying psychological and sociological determinants are responsible for the development and perpetuation of the disorder (Balis, 1974). Therefore, detoxification is not a rehabilitative procedure but rather a prerequisite for accomplishing the goal of rehabilitation. It serves as a stepping stone that may

permit entry of the patient into more definitive treatment (see treatment of Substance Use Disorders).

The following general principles are based on guidelines and procedures established by the National Institute on Drug Abuse (Czechowicz, 1978).

A thorough evaluation of the patient should serve as the cornerstone for developing an appropriate treatment plan for detoxification. This involves:

1) identification of the drugs used and assessment of the level of tolerance to and the degree of physical dependence on each;
2) medical history with a thorough review of systems;
3) psychiatric history and mental status examination;
4) physical examination; and
5) appropriate laboratory tests.

The decision regarding appropriate locus of detoxification (inpatient, outpatient, residential) involves a number of considerations including type of substance dependence, available resources, and the individual's life-style. In general, opiate detoxification can be done in an outpatient or residential setting. Alcohol detoxification should generally be conducted in a hospital or emergency room setting; however, patients with mild-to-moderate withdrawal reactions can be managed at home or in a specialized residential setting. Barbiturate-type, meprobamate, and/or polydrug dependence require a hospital setting in order to prevent life-threatening complications. Amphetamine withdrawal may require hospitalization in the presence of significant suicidal risk. The patient should participate voluntarily (and sign an informed consent) unless he/she is incompetent, as in the case of an intervening delirium. The staff should be familiar with laws regulating the use and disclosure of information about patients undergoing treatment for substance abuse.

A detoxification treatment plan should follow certain general guidelines:

(a) Whenever possible a long-acting drug should be substituted for a short-acting drug of addiction.
(b) The initial amount of the drug required to suppress withdrawal symptoms is determined empirically, by assessing symptom response to repeated drug dosages (e.g., alcohol withdrawal) or through a challenge test (e.g., barbiturate withdrawal).
(c) The detoxification procedure should be safe and geared to provide a comfortable withdrawal through individualized titration and progressive withdrawal of the drug.

(d) The patient should be closely monitored for signs and symptoms of withdrawal or intoxication as a means of titrating dosage and pace of withdrawal schedule.

(e) Upon completion of the detoxification procedure, provision should be made for an aftercare plan with appropriate referral for further treatment and rehabilitation (except in the case of accidental or iatrogenic dependence).

SPECIFIC DISORDERS

291.80   Alcohol Withdrawal
291.00   Alcohol Withdrawal Delirium
The severity of the withdrawal depends on the amount, frequency, and duration of prior alcohol consumption. It is usually benign and self-limited, unless it progresses to a Withdrawal Delirium. Alcohol Withdrawal Delirium (delirium tremens) is a serious withdrawal complication occurring in about 5% of the cases and occasionally leading to death from intercurrent illness (Victor & Adams, 1953).

Patients with Withdrawal Delirium, as well as those with severe withdrawal syndrome, must be hospitalized, preferably in a special detoxification unit. After medical evaluation (especially for subdural hematoma, pancreatitis, infections, hepatic disease, and malnutrition), treatment should include the following:

(a) The patient should be sedated with a benzodiazepine (chlordiazepoxide, diazepam) as the drug of choice (Greenblatt & Shader, 1975; Sellers & Kalant, 1976). Neuroleptics, paraldehyde, and magnesium sulfate have also been successfully used. Barbiturates, although effective, should be avoided. Chlordiazepoxide 25–50 mg or diazepam 5–10 mg may be given orally or intramuscularly and repeated every two to four hours as necessary until symptoms are suppressed, and then reduced to half that dose three or four times per day orally. In impending or acute withdrawal delirium, the slow intravenous administration of these drugs is preferred because the intramuscular route is slow and unpredictable. Benzodiazepines and paraldehyde provide an anticonvulsant effect, thus reducing the risk of withdrawal seizures. Neuroleptics, on the other hand, tend to increase the risk of developing convulsions. Magnesium sulfate has been used by some in patients with low serum magnesium (below 2 mEq/L). It is given intravenously in a 5% solution in doses up to 2.0 gm, repeated three to four times daily for three days and then reduced to 1.0 gm daily for an additional two to three days (Mendelson, 1970; Stending-Lindberg, 1974).

(b) The patient should be given thiamine (initial dose of 100–200 mg I.M., with subsequent doses given orally) and a multi-vitamin supplement, to combat malnutrition and prevent acute thiamine deficiency that may lead to Wernicke-Korsakoff Amnestic Syndrome or cardiac failure (Cade, 1970).

(c) Parenteral fluid administration should be carefully individualized and titrated according to the hydration status of the patient. Fluid retention and overhydration develop during rising blood alcohol levels, while dehydration follows a period of stable high blood alcohol levels. Therefore, many patients may actually be overhydrated, in which case parenteral fluids are contraindicated (Ogata et al., 1968). Dehydration is presumed in cases of vomiting, diarrhea, elevated hematocrit and other objective signs of dehydration. No more than 50% of an initial fluid deficit should be replaced during the first 24 hours, and no more than 6 liters of dextrose-containing fluid should be given in a 24-hour period (Czechowicz, 1978). Fluids should be given orally if the patient is not severely ill and can tolerate oral intake. Any electrolyte deficit should be corrected.

(d) Hypoglycemia may be present in some patients during the withdrawal period. Patients should be given a sufficient amount of carbohydrate in oral fluids (e.g., orange juice). Parenteral fluids, if needed, should contain 5% dextrose (Freinkel & Arky, 1966).

(e) Alcohol withdrawal seizures (grand mal) are generally self-limited and have a relatively benign course. There is no evidence that prophylactic use of phenytoin (Dilantin) will prevent withdrawal seizures. Benzodiazepines are effective in lessening the likelihood of seizures and will suffice for the patient who has no history of epilepsy. Prophylactic anticonvulsant therapy is indicated in patients known to have an underlying seizure disorder. In the event that withdrawal seizures occur, diazepam 5–10 mg slow I.V. is recommended (Czechowicz, 1978).

(f) Concurrent disorders (e.g., gastritis, pancreatitis, anemia) may also require proper evaluation and treatment.

General management of the delirious patient is discussed in the section on Delirium.

292.00   Barbiturate or Similarly Acting Sedative or
          Hypnotic Withdrawal
292.00   Barbiturate or Similarly Acting Sedative or
          Hypnotic Withdrawal Delirium

Barbiturate and similarly acting sedative or hypnotic drugs (ethchlorvynol, glutethimide, methyprylon, chloral hydrate, paraldehyde, methaqualone, meprobamate, and benzodiazepines) produce a withdrawal syndrome almost identical to that of alcohol. Threshold doses and time periods necessary for development of physical dependence vary according to the type of drug used. Daily doses of 900 mg or more of pentobarbital for one-to-two months will lead, upon sudden withdrawal, to convulsions in 75 % of subjects and to delirium in 65 % (Fraser et al., 1964). Barbiturate withdrawal will begin 12–24 hours after the last dose was taken. Grand mal seizures most often occur between the third and seventh day and may lead to status epilepticus. The withdrawal delirium most often occurs between the fourth and sixth day. Hyperpyrexia, cardiovascular collapse, and death may occur in untreated cases. Convulsions associated with benzodiazepine withdrawal syndrome may appear several weeks after the discontinuation of the drug.

Detoxification of patients with barbiturate or similarly-acting substance dependence should generally be carried out in a hospital setting. These patients need very close medical supervision because of the life-threatening nature of the abstinence syndrome. Detoxification is accomplished by the use of one of the following procedures: (a) phenobarbital substitution; (b) pentobarbital substitution; or (c) slow withdrawal of the addicting agent (Czechowicz, 1978).

Phenobarbital Substitution. The stabilization dose of phenobarbital to be given daily is tentatively calculated on the basis of the patient's history and by monitoring the patient's response to the drug. The initial daily requirement is calculated by substituting one sedative dose (30 mg) of phenobarbital for each hypnotic dose of any reported sedative-hypnotic. The equivalent of 30 mg of phenobarbital for short-acting barbiturates (amobarbital, pentobarbital, secobarbital) is about 100 mg; for chloral hydrate, 500 mg; for ethclorvynol, 350 mg; for glutethimide, 250 mg; for meprobamate, 400–600 mg; for methaqualone, 250–200 mg; and for methyprylon, 300 mg (Smith & Wesson, 1970). *The initial total daily dose of phenobarbital should never exceed 600 mg, regardless of the dosage claimed by the patient.* The established daily requirement is given in divided doses, three or four times daily. If toxic symptoms occur (slurred speech, nystagmus, ataxia), the daily dose should be reduced. The patient should be maintained on the stabilization dosage for two days before graded withdrawal is initiated. Once this is achieved, the total daily dose of phenobarbital is reduced by 30 mg per day. During this period, the patient should be closely monitored for signs of withdrawal of phenobarbital toxicity so that the dosage can be titrated accordingly.

Pentobarbital Substitution. This method is used in cases involving dependence on a short-acting barbiturate. A short-acting barbiturate (pentobarbital) is employed for substitution. The initial daily requirement is calculated by the use of the pentobarbital challenge test. This test helps to establish the degree of barbiturate tolerance (and thus dependence) through the repeated administration of a standard dose of 200 mg of pentobarbital at two-hour intervals until signs of barbiturate toxicity are elicited. The patient is first given 200 mg of pentobarbital orally. If he/she does not show any signs of intoxication (e.g., nystagmus, unsteady gait, slurred speech) after two hours, the dose is repeated. No further treatment is necessary if a dose of 400 mg or less results in intoxication. If no signs of intoxication are present, it is assumed that the individual demonstrated tolerance and physical dependence, and therefore needs detoxification. The next step involves the estimation of the daily barbiturate requirement for that individual by continuing the challenge test until signs of mild intoxication are produced. The total amount of pentobarbital given becomes the stabilization dosage level. After a two-day period of stabilization the pentobarbital is gradually withdrawn by 10% of the total drug dosage per day, not to exceed 100 mg per day. Rate and amount of reduction may need to be adjusted if withdrawal signs occur.

Slow Withdrawal of the Addicting Agent. This method is applied in patients dependent on benzodiazepines, long-acting sedative hypnotics, or mixed sedative hypnotics. Initially, the patient is given the addicting drug at the dosage level of his/her daily intake and then he/she is gradually withdrawn from it at a daily decreasing rate of about 20% of the total dosage per day (Hollister et al., 1966; Khantziam & McKenna, 1979).

In the case of barbiturate withdrawal delirium, the patient should be sedated to the point of mild intoxication and be stabilized (suppression of all withdrawal symptoms) for two days before detoxification is started. In extreme agitation, the initial dose of the sedative is given intravenously (e.g., diazepam 10 mg, or amobarbital 500 mg) (Wulff, 1959).

292.00 Opioid Withdrawal

The time of onset and duration of the syndrome vary depending on the action of the drug used (e.g., shortest course with hydromorphone, and longest with methadone). Heroin and morphine withdrawal syndrome begins 8–12 hours following last dose and gradually subsides over a period of 7–10 days. Evidence of dependence may be demonstrated by the naloxone test: Intramuscular injection of 0.4 mg of naloxone (Narcan) will precipitate withdrawal symptoms in an opioid dependent individual.

Detoxification from opioids can be carried out in an inpatient, residential, or outpatient setting. The following procedure describes management in a hospital setting. Pretreatment evaluation includes a complete medical and drug abuse history, physical examination, routine laboratory tests, and urine screening for drugs of abuse. Following verification of opioid dependence, the patient is treated by the method of methadone substitution. The standard approach is to give an initial dose of 10–20 mg of oral methadone. If withdrawal symptoms are not suppressed, an additional 5–10 mg of methadone may be given. The total dose for the day should not exceed 40 mg. Once the stabilizing dosage is estimated, the patient is maintained on that level for two or three days, with methadone given once a day or in b.i.d. divided doses. Detoxification then begins with a reduction each day by 15–20% of the total methadone daily dose (usually about 5 mg per day). The withdrawal is completed in 7–10 days.

Detoxification of individuals on methadone maintenance requires prior confirmation of maintenance dosage and enrollment in a methadone maintenance program. In these patients the detoxification period should last longer, extending several weeks, at a rate of reduction of 3–5 mg per day. It is generally recommended that withdrawal from methadone maintenance be conducted on an outpatient basis by a process of gradual detoxification over a period of four-to-six months, with a dose decrement of approximately 3% per week.

Recent reports have documented the effectiveness of the antihypertensive clonidine for suppressing the symptoms of opioid withdrawal (Charney et al., 1981; Gold et al., 1980; Washton & Resnick, 1980). More information is needed regarding optimal doses and administration schedules.

292.00 Amphetamine or Similarly Acting Sympathomimetic Withdrawal

The syndrome may progress during the first two weeks to a major depression involving significant suicidal risk, which may persist for months. In view of the suicidal risk involved, detoxification from amphetamines should be carried out in a controlled environment and under close observation, preferably in a psychiatric hospital setting. The addicting drug should be promptly discontinued and the patient placed on suicide precautions. If the patient is severely agitated or psychotic (see Intoxication, Delirium, and Organic Delusional Syndrome) upon admission, he/she may be treated initially with moderate doses of a neuroleptic, which should be tapered and discontinued upon control of the target symptoms. If the syndrome develops into a depressive episode, treatment with antidepressants may be necessary, following the guidelines applicable to depressive disorders. In the presence of a concurrent delusional syndrome, tricyclic treatment should be combined with the administration of neuroleptics. Psychotherapeutic management and psychosocial counseling should be provided, as well as referral to a treatment program prior to discharge (Berger & Tinklenberg, 1979; Ellinwood, 1979).

292.00   Tobacco Withdrawal
Management of Tobacco Withdrawal is discussed in the section on Substance Use Disorders.

Mixed Drug Withdrawal
In mixed substance dependencies, detoxification should proceed with the gradual withdrawal of one drug at a time, while stabilizing the patient on the other drug(s) on which he or she may be dependent.

In the instance of combined heroin and barbiturate dependence, it is preferable to withdraw the barbiturate first, while stabilizing the patient on methadone. Following withdrawal from the barbiturate, one may proceed with detoxification from the opioid (Czechowicz, 1978).

In the instance of alcohol-barbiturate dependence, the detoxification procedure is similar to other sedative-hypnotic dependence, since the substances have an additive effect. One must calculate the phenobarbital equivalent of alcohol (15 mg phenobarbital for 1 ounce of 80–100 proof alcohol) and add it to the phenobarbital equivalent of the sedative hypnotic (Czechowicz, 1978).

In the instance of opiate-alcohol dependence, it is preferable to begin with the alcohol detoxification, while stabilizing the patient on methadone, and then proceed with methadone withdrawal (Czechowicz, 1978).

INTOXICATIONS
Intoxication represents poisoning by a substance that directly affects the CNS, producing substance-specific mental disturbances associated with maladaptive behavior. Substance-specific physiological disturbances may lead to serious medical complications including cardiopulmonary impairment, coma, or death. The severity of the syndrome is generally dose-related, although, in some instances, it may be idiosyncratic in nature (e.g., pathological alcohol intoxication).

General Therapeutic Principles
The following review will focus on the treatment and management of acute episodes of intoxication that involve overdosage with drugs of abuse. The treatment of Substance Use Disorders will be discussed in a separate chapter.

The following general principles are applicable to all cases of acute, severe intoxications seen in the Emergency Room of a hospital (Czechowicz, 1978).

1) Upon admission of the intoxicated patient, determine immediately the adequacy of cardiopulmonary functions and level of consciousness. Begin cardiopulmonary resuscitation and other life support at once, if needed (see #4 below).

2) Establish a working diagnosis on the basis of available information and clinical evidence. Of immediate concern are the identification of the substance used, its route of entry into the body, and its amount. In addition to the history and physical examination, institute urine and blood screening for drugs and other laboratory tests as appropriate to evaluate the nature and seriousness of the intoxication.

3) Apply measures to eliminate the toxic substance from the body, if needed. In cases of ingested substances in which the overdose occurred within the preceding six hours, immediate measures may include induced emesis, gastric lavage, activated charcoal, and cathartics. Induced vomiting is contraindicated in the presence of impaired consciousness or convulsions. Emesis may be induced with ipecac syrup 30–45 ml; this dose may be repeated in 15 minutes if necessary. Gastric lavage requires prior endotracheal intubation in a patient who has evidence of CNS depression; it is contraindicated if the patient is convulsing. After lavage is completed, introduce activated charcoal into the stomach to absorb any remaining drug. The use of cathartics (e.g., 30 cc of sorbitol or 30 mg of sodium sulfate) is not a well established procedure (Davis & Benvenuto, 1975).

Later, if toxic drug levels persist, it may become necessary to apply other measures for the elimination of the substance, for instance by increasing urinary excretion or by the use of aqueous or lipid dialysis (peritoneal lavage or hemodialysis). Increased urinary excretion of the substance may be accomplished by administering sufficient fluids to promote urine output, by forced diuresis with I.V. 20% mannitol at the rate of 50 cc per hour or by the alkalinization of the urine with sodium bicarbonate, as in phenobarbital poisoning.

4) Apply measures that reduce the toxic physiologic effects of the substance, as needed. Prompt treatment of impaired vital functions (support of respiration and blood pressure) takes precedence over any other intervention. Assure a clear airway and administer oxygen, if necessary. Provide mechanical ventilation by ambu bag or positive pressure respirator if respiration is not present, and then proceed with endotracheal intubation. Rarely, tracheotomy may be necessary. Start I.V. fluids to maintain blood pressure; vasopressors may be used if fluid therapy fails to restore blood pressure. Upon sta-

bilization of vital functions, obtain an EKG to detect cardiac arrhythmias and provide treatment if necessary.

In every stuporous or comatose patient, the glucose-naloxone test should be administered routinely as a means of ruling out hypoglycemic or opioid-induced coma: Administer intravenously 50 cc of 50% glucose and 0.4 mg naloxone (Narcan). Both agents are safe and readily reverse the respective hypoglycemic or opioid-induced coma. Physostigmine (1–2 mg I.V.) may serve as an antidote to anticholinergic coma; if successful, it will require frequent repeating. Symptomatic treatment may also control seizures, hyperthermia, cardiac arrhythmias, and so forth.

5) Adequacy of treatment should be regularly assessed by monitoring vital signs, arterial blood gases, drug blood levels, and level of consciousness. Continuous EKG monitoring may be necessary in intoxication with cardiotoxic drugs (e.g., tricyclics).

6) In less serious intoxications, the concomitant behavioral disturbances (agitation, combativeness, suicidal attempts) may become the major focus of management. One may first place the patient in a quiet room and secure his or her safety (as well as that of the attending staff) by providing constant supervision and, if necessary, applying physical restraint. Sedation may be required for the excited or violent patient, but must be used cautiously. In the case of the "bad tripper" (e.g., Hallucinogen Hallucinosis, Cannabis Delusional Disorder), the "talk-down" method is the most important aspect of management (see respective sections).

More complete discussion of management of medical emergencies is beyond the scope of this book.

SPECIFIC DISORDERS

303.00   Alcohol Intoxication
Most cases of Alcohol Intoxication do not require any special treatment. The most common problem requiring management is combative or assaultive behavior and, occasionally, suicidal behavior. The patient should be handled with a non-provocative, reassuring approach. Physical restraint may become necessary in combative individuals. The use of sedative drugs should be avoided because of their potentiating effects with alcohol. The least dangerous drug is chlordiazepoxide, which may be used cautiously as a chemical restraint in parenteral doses of 50–100 mg. In more severe intoxications, the CNS depressant effects of alcohol may impair vital functions (see General Therapeutic Principles in section on Intoxications). If there is evidence of recent drug use, gastric lavage and other symptomatic treatment may become

necessary. In the case of alcohol-disulfiram interaction, treatment consists of the I.V. administration of an antihistamine and symptomatic control of hypotension.

291.40 Alcohol Idiosyncratic Intoxication

This consists of marked behavioral change—usually aggressiveness—resulting from the recent ingestion of a subintoxicating amount of alcohol. Brain damage and temporal lobe epilepsy are considered to be predisposing factors. Treatment is primarily directed toward the management of aggressive or assaultive behavior.

305.40 Barbiturate or Similarly Acting Sedative or Hypnotic Intoxication

In mild-to-moderate sedative-hypnotic intoxication, if the patient is conscious and ambulatory, the management is primarily directed to monitoring the vital signs and controlling agitation or aggressiveness. The patient should be placed in a quiet room under close supervision; the use of physical restraint may become necessary in the presence of combativeness. In more serious intoxications, treatment largely consists of supportive care and maintenance of vital functions (see General Therapeutic Principles section on Intoxications). In overdose of short-acting barbiturates, forced diuresis is of no value. On the other hand, forced diuresis (e.g., I.V. 20% mannitol at a rate of 50 cc per hour) can be very effective in meprobamate overdosage. Urine alkalinization with sodium bicarbonate can be helpful in phenobarbital overdosage, by increasing the urinary excretion of the drug. In overdose of nonbarbiturate sedative-hypnotics, forced diuresis and dialysis may be useful for certain drugs when response to other measures is unsatisfactory (Czechowicz, 1978). Aqueous dialysis is of little value in glutethimide poisoning, because of the drug's protein binding and storage in body fat (Davis & Benvenuto, 1975). Glutethimide overdose may cause a coma-wakefulness cycle by means of excretion into and reabsorption from the G.I. tract. Gastric lavage, if performed, should be done with a 1 : 1 mixture of castor oil and water. If hemodialysis is attempted, it should involve a lipid dialysate (Lewis & Senay, 1981). In methaqualone overdose, the presence of an intact gag reflex may present difficulties during endotracheal intubation; dialysis may be helpful.

305.50 Opioid Intoxication

In more serious opioid poisoning, medical complications include depressed respiration, depressed consciousness, hypotension, and pulmonary edema. Instead of myosis, pupils may be dilated in cases with severe hypoxia or in mixed addictions. Meperidine may cause dilated pupils and is more frequently associated with convulsions. Heroin may remain active for six hours, methadone for 36–48 hours, and l-alpha-acetyl-methadol (LAAM) for 48–72 hours (Berger & Tinklenberg, 1979; Czechowicz, 1978; Lewis & Senay, 1981).

Management of the acute opioid intoxication involves prompt treatment of respiratory impairment and maintenance of vital functions (see General Therapeutic Principles for Intoxications). Naloxone (Narcan) 0.4 mg I.V. is effective in reversing both respiratory depression and coma. If the initial dose is ineffective, an additional dose may be given in about five minutes and again in 10 minutes. Failure to respond should raise consideration of other causes for the intoxication (Czechowicz, 1978). Narcotic antagonists are effective for about two to three hours; therefore, repeat doses may be necessary at regular intervals to continue to reverse respiratory depression. If withdrawal symptoms are precipitated, they should not be treated with methadone. The patient should remain hospitalized under continuous supervision for 24–48 hours. If pulmonary edema occurs, the treatment of choice is oxygen administration, with positive pressure ventilation and intubation, if necessary (Czechowicz, 1978).

305.60   Cocaine Intoxication
305.70   Amphetamine or Similarly Acting Sympathomimetic Intoxication

Medical complications in acute overdose consist of severe hypertension, hyperpyrexia, seizures, syncope, cardiac arrhythmias or respiratory paralysis. Cocaine and amphetamine-like drugs produce very similar intoxication syndromes.

An initial characteristic "rush" of well-being is followed after one hour or longer by a period of "crashing." A suicidal depression may ensue as a complication of withdrawal (see Amphetamine Withdrawal Syndrome).

The management of a mild-to-moderate psychostimulant intoxication syndrome requires placement of the patient in a quiet room where safety measures may be applied for the protection of the patient and the attending staff. If reassurance is not sufficient to calm the patient, sedation with benzodiazepines (e.g., diazepam 10–30 mg orally) may control agitation. Physical restraint may become necessary to control combativeness. Vital signs should be monitored closely for rising blood pressure, pulse, and temperature. In acute overdose, treatment with neuroleptics is recommended when blood pressure, pulse rate, or temperature is rising, or if acute paranoid behavior develops, provided that no anticholinergic drugs were involved in the intoxication. It should be noted that chlorpromazine, although an effective antidote, has strong anticholinergic effects. The drug of choice is haloperidol, given in an initial dose of 3–5 mg P.O. or I.M., with subsequent doses adjusted to the need for controlling the above symptoms (Davis et al., 1973). Uncontrollable severe hypertension should be treated with intravenous phentolamine, while hyperpyrexia should be treated with the standard medical techniques. Increased fluids and acidification of urine with ammonium chloride can significantly enhance the excretion of the drug (Berger & Tinklenberg, 1979). If psychosis and elevated vital signs persist in spite of adequate treatment, the patient requires hospitalization. Consideration should be given to the possibility of suicidal depression that may develop during Amphetamine Withdrawal or persistent psychosis associated with the Amphetamine Delusional Syndrome (Berger & Tinklenberg, 1979; Ellinwood, 1979). Amphetamine Delirium has already been discussed elsewhere.

305.20 Cannabis Intoxication
In moderate doses cannabis acts as a sedative drug, while at high doses it acts as a hallucinogen. Hashish, hash oil, and tetrahydrocannabinol (THC) are much more potent than cannabis and are more likely to induce Cannabis Hallucinosis. The latter, however, is very rare.

Cannabis Intoxication is relatively mild and short-lived and does not generally require treatment intervention. Acute panic associated with Cannabis Intoxication is generally managed by the "talking-down" approach, already described in Hallucinogen Hallucinosis. The treatment of Cannabis Delusional Disorder has also been discussed elsewhere.

305.90 Phencyclidine (PCP) or Similarly Acting
Arylcyclohexylamine Intoxication
Severe PCP intoxication is characterized by motor inhibition and catatonic-like states, stupor, or coma with the eyes remaining open, seizures, opisthotonos, hyperreflexia, severe hypertension, and respiratory depression. Bloody vomiting should suggest possible contamination by a synthetic intermediate which decomposes to yield hydrogen cyanide. The absence of mydriasis and the presence of ataxia, hypertension, and nystagmus differentiate PCP intoxication from hallucinogen intoxication (Lewis & Senay, 1981). Delirium and Mixed Organic Mental Disorder may develop.

In low-dose intoxication, the key to management is sensory reduction and protection from self-harm. The patient should be kept in a quiet room, closely supervised from a distance. Physical restraint may be necessary if violent behavior occurs. For sedation, diazepam or haloperidol are the drugs of choice. In moderate to severe intoxication, close observation with monitoring of blood pressure, respiration, and level of consciousness is required. If serious hypertension develops, diazoxide and hydralazine have been reported to be effective in lowering blood pressure (Lewis & Senay, 1981). If status epilepticus develops, diazepam in 2-3 mg increments slow I.V. is indicated. Acidification of the urine with ammonium chloride markedly enhances PCP excretion (Aniline et al., 1981). Continuous or intermittent gastric suction has been recommended as a means of enhancing PCP excretion (Lewis & Senay, 1981). Prolonged psychotic reactions following PCP intoxication are discussed in the section on Organic Delusional Syndromes.

305.90   Caffeine Intoxication

Toxic symptoms subside rapidly after reduction of intake or abstinence. Transient mild withdrawal symptoms may occur in chronic heavy users. No pharmacologic treatment is necessary. Massive overdose may result in seizures that can be controlled with I.V. diazepam. The substitution of a decaffeinated beverage may prove helpful to some (Greden, 1980).

305.90   Anticholinergic Drug Intoxication

This type of intoxication is of particular interest because of the widespread use of substances with anticholinergic activity. Intoxication is characterized by: (a) dilated and unreactive pupils, flushed face, warm and dry skin, dry mouth, paralytic ileus, urinary retention, tachycardia, hypertension or hypotension, increased respiratory rate, seizures, hyperpyrexia; and (b) delirium, hallucinations, delusions, severe agitation and assaultiveness, stupor and coma. In addition to the above, the comatose patient may show hyperreflexia, positive Babinski's sign, and clonic movements (Berger & Tinklenberg, 1979; Goldfrank & Meliek, 1979; Granacher et al., 1976). Cardiotoxic effects with tricyclics include, in addition to the supraventricular tachycardia, ventricular tachyarrhythmias, cardiac conduction defects and A/V block, and direct suppression of the myocardium (Goldfrank & Meliek, 1979; Granacher et al., 1976).

Patient management includes the usual measures for overdosage (emesis, gastric lavage, maintenance of cardiopulmonary functions, monitoring of vital signs) and symptomatic treatment of anticholinergic effects. Physostigmine salicylate 2 mg I.V. is capable of reversing the coma, and controlling delirium, hyperthermia, and supraventricular tachycardia secondary to anticholinergic toxicity (Heizer & Wilbert, 1974). A second dose of 1-2 mg physostigmine may be given 15 minutes later, and it may be repeated every two to three hours, if needed. Close monitoring of anticholinergic symptoms is required.

Cholinergic toxicity induced by overmedication with physostigmine can be reversed by atropine 0.1 to 1.0 mg I.V. or propantheline bromide (Proban-thine) 15–30 mg I.M. or I.V. (Lewis & Senay, 1981).

Agitation in milder cases may be controlled with diazepam, provided that vital functions are stable and the patient is fully conscious. Seizures can be controlled with intravenous diazepam. Cardiac arrhythmias, other than supraventricular tachycardia, are treated with intravenous fluids and alka-linization with sodium bicarbonate or sodium lactate; if there is no improve-ment, propranolol and lidocaine can be useful. Prolonged EKG monitoring is extremely important for diagnosing cardiac arrhythmias, and as a means of assessing severity of intoxication. The latter correlates with the degree of widening of QRS complex and prolongation of QT interval (Goldfrank & Meliek, 1979; Granacher et al., 1976).

Chapter 3

Substance Use Disorders

Substance Abuse is distinguished from non-pathological substance use by: (a) a pattern of pathological use; (b) impairment in social or occupational functioning caused by the pattern of pathological use; and (c) duration of at least one month. *Substance Dependence* is a more severe form of Substance Abuse that is accompanied by physical dependence, evidenced by either tolerance or withdrawal. The course of Substance Use Disorders may be continuous, episodic, or in remission. Early detection and treatment are crucial for the optimal prognosis of these disorders.

Personality disturbance and other psychopathology (e.g., depression, anxiety) are often present as associated features. Higher incidence of psychopathology is found among the polydrug abusers than in individuals abusing a single drug. Complications resulting from Substance Abuse or Substance Dependence include: (a) substance-specific Organic Brain Syndromes; (b) deterioration of physical health due to malnutrition and poor hygiene; (c) medical complications due to the effects of the substance (e.g., cirrhosis, peripheral neuropathy, acute pancreatitis associated with Alcohol Dependence), or due to the administration of the substance by contaminated needles (e.g., hepatitis, vasculitis, septicemia in Opioid Dependence); and (d) depressive symptoms that partly account for the high rate of suicide by individuals with Substance Dependence.

GENERAL THERAPEUTIC PRINCIPLES

The field is replete with treatment approaches, based on diverse theories and ideologies, with claims of therapeutic successes that generally lack objective substantiation. The following principles constitute general guidelines that should be taken into consideration in formulating a treatment and management plan.

1) There is not any singular treatment modality that can claim high effectiveness for chemical dependence.

2) A combination of modalities must be used in order to achieve a measure of therapeutic success.

3) Choice of treatment modalities must be tailored to the individual, taking into consideration his or her specific problems, response to previous treatment attempts, and the resources available.

4) Different treatment and management approaches are administered by a great variety of professionals, nonprofessional practitioners, and lay groups. The physician plays a central role in the initial evaluation and medical diagnosis, management of physical-psychiatric complications, detoxification, and appropriate referral. In follow-up care, the general physician may apply some of the specific methods available, or may collaborate with other practitioners and various agencies involved in the treatment and rehabilitation of the patient.

5) A prerequisite for any treatment plan is the detoxification of the patient (see Treatment section on Withdrawal and Withdrawal Deliria).

6) The presence of associated psychopathology requires specialized psychiatric treatment, especially with regard to affective disorders and personality disorders (e.g., antisocial, borderline).

7) The socially dislocated individual (e.g., unemployed, homeless, legally entangled, or culturally alienated) requires social and vocational rehabilitation, with the goal of reintegrating him or her into his or her family, community, or work setting.

Treatment modalities that are currently available include the following:

1) *Pharmacologic methods,* such as disulfiram for alcoholism, narcotic maintenance and narcotic antagonists for opioid dependence, and various psychotropic drugs for the short-term management of targeted symptoms of anxiety and depression following detoxification.

2) *Psychosocial methods* including individual psychotherapy, group therapy, family therapy, conjoint therapy with spouse, psychodrama, behavior modification, aversive conditioning, and relaxation techniques.

3) *Sociotherapies,* such as various therapeutic communities (e.g., Synanon) and other residential programs (e.g., halfway houses).

4) *Self-support groups,* such as Alcoholics Anonymous, Al-Anon, Alateen, Narcotics Anonymous.

5) *Various therapeutic, educational, occupational, inspirational, or humane programs,* supported or sponsored by government agencies, industry, religious organizations (e.g., Salvation Army), and other community and volunteer agencies.

Common factors that appear to contribute to the therapeutic success of most effective treatment modalities include the following:

1) Patience, perseverance, and commitment on the part of the therapist while working with a very difficult and frustrating patient who is suffering from a chronic and relapsing disorder. This should be laced with a hopeful expectation, kindled by a caring and nurturing but firm attitude, tempered by a realistic appraisal of the patient's potential and limitations, and monitored by an awareness of transference-countertransference problems.

2) Maintenance of abstinence during treatment and the setting of abstinence as the ultimate treatment goal.

3) A degree of coerciveness that ranges from subtle measures of substance control to coercion by commitment to a treatment facility. Thus, coerciveness may take the form of "contracts" that the patient is persuaded or often forced to make with the therapist, spouse, or employer, in the face of crisis situations. Structured environments, disulfiram administered under supervision, or limit-setting in therapy for acting out are other examples of coerciveness.

4) Breaking through the defense of massive denial. A major effort during the initial phase of treatment is to help the patient to recognize and accept the problem.

5) Maintenance of the patient's wavering motivation to stay in treatment and remain abstinent.

6) Development of alternative coping styles to handle intense dysphoric affects, especially with regard to rage, guilt, anxiety, and depression; boosting and maintenance of self-esteem; and controlling various environmental contingencies and social stimulus factors in drug effects.

SPECIFIC DISORDERS

305.0x   Alcohol Abuse
303.9x   Alcohol Dependence
Detoxification is the first step before treatment of alcoholism is undertaken. Detoxification and treatment of psychiatric complications of alcoholism (Or-

ganic Brain Syndromes) were discussed elsewhere (see Treatment of Organic Mental Disorders).

A comprehensive multiple treatment approach is the best basic premise for treating alcoholism. Several treatment modalities should be integrated in a treatment plan that is tailored to the particular needs of the individual and the resources available. The usual treatment plan includes psychotherapy (individual or group therapy and conjoint therapy if the patient is married), disulfiram, and short-term use of tranquilizers or antidepressants for targeted symptoms (Gerard & Saenger, 1966). The patient should be urged to join Alcoholics Anonymous and attend meetings regularly. Al-Anon provides assistance to spouses of alcoholics through group support, while Alateen serves the needs of children of alcoholic parents. Referral of members of the family of the alcoholic to these organizations should be part of the multiple treatment approach.

Halfway houses may serve as an important treatment resource for patients with domiciliary placement problems following detoxification and discharge from the hospital. Referral to vocational rehabilitation and social support agencies may be required for selected cases (Selzer, 1980). In most communities, there are comprehensive alcoholism treatment and rehabilitation programs in which a multiple modality treatment approach is available. Specialized residential treatment may be necessary for some patients.

The primary physician plays a crucial role in the diagnosis and treatment of the alcoholic patient. Dealing with the patient's denial is an early and decisive task (Whitfield, 1982). One strategy is to give the patient the Michigan Alcoholism Screening Test (MAST) which has proved to be a reliable and valid test for diagnosing alcoholism (Selzer et al., 1975). An authoritative demonstration of the problem may serve as the first step in loosening up the patient's defensive armor. With acceptance of the problem and the establishment of a therapeutic alliance, the physician can proceed with the task of negotiating a "therapeutic contract" with the patient (Brady et al., 1982).

Long-term abstinence should be the goal. If this is not possible, a trial period of abstinence is an acceptable compromise. The contract should include means of deterrence to drinking and ways of monitoring compliance. The use of disulfiram (Antabuse) as a temporary deterrent against impulsive drinking is very helpful. A challenge dose of alcohol after disulfiram is begun is not necessary, provided the patient is fully instructed about the consequences of drinking within four days of ingestion of the drug. Disulfiram is given at bedtime in a loading dose of 500 mg daily for five to seven days, then continued on a daily maintenance dose of 250 mg. A spouse or some other person should be involved in administering the disulfiram at least every three or four days to ensure compliance. Another method is to contract with the patient to visit briefly with the therapist every three or four days during the first month for monitoring the actual taking of the drug (Goodwin, 1982). During these brief visits the emphasis is on talking about problems most alcoholics face when they stop drinking. After the month is over, a new contract is negotiated, with the patient assuming responsibility for control of his drinking (Goodwin, 1982).

The psychotherapeutic approach is primarily supportive with many of these patients; the therapist plays an active and nurturing role while maintaining clear boundaries of separateness and setting firm limits that discourage acting out. Behavior therapy techniques for behavior modification, relaxation, assertiveness training, self-control skills, aversive conditioning, and biofeedback have become part of some alcoholism treatment programs.

Benzodiazepines and small doses of neuroleptics are recommended for short-term use following detoxification, given on an as needed basis for control of anxiety (Rothstein et al., 1976). The development of depression may require treatment with tricyclic antidepressants.

305.5x   Opioid Abuse
304.0x   Opioid Dependence

Treatment programs for the opioid abuser (mainly heroin) include methadone maintenance, maintenance with opioid antagonists, therapeutic communities, drug-free programs, and detoxification programs. Most of these provide a combination of adjunctive approaches, such as group therapy for improvement of social skills, vocational training, job placement, and family counseling.

Methadone maintenance is the most common and most successful treatment for opioid dependence (Mirin & Meyer, 1978). It is offered in special clinics under close supervision and monitoring. Unlike heroin, methadone is long-acting (24 hours), and is orally effective. In usual doses (40–50 mg), it blocks opioid craving, while in much higher doses (100–120 mg) it even blocks the euphoriant effects of opioids. The most significant effect for maintenance is the blocking of opioid craving (Goldstein & Judson, 1973). In spite of some criticism, methadone maintenance is an effective and safe method that allows the opioid addict to change his or her life-style and reintegrate into the community. Treatment goals are reduction of illicit drug use, reduction of criminal activity, increased employability, increased self-esteem, and improvement in family and community functioning (Berger & Tinklenberg, 1979; Green et al., 1975; Kissin et al., 1978). According to FDA regulations, those eligible for methadone maintenance are individuals whose dependence on heroin has lasted longer than two years. It is indicated for addicts who are not strongly motivated to achieve immediate abstinence. A typical methadone maintenance clinic provides daily administration of oral methadone, monitored with urinalysis, plus counseling and ancillary services, and group therapy. The most common complication in methadone-monitored patients is alcoholism (O'Donnell, 1969). Levo-alpha-acetylmethadol (LAAM) is a long-acting congener of methadone, currently under investigational trials, which can be administered three times per week, thus affording greater treatment flexibility (Ling & Blaine, 1979).

Maintenance with opioid antagonists is currently undergoing field trials as a new treatment approach. Its goal is to decondition the behaviors of opioid use and relapse (Whitlock & Evans, 1978). By blocking both the euphoria and the relief of conditioned abstinence symptoms of the former opioid abuser, narcotic antagonists may help extinguish the behaviors of opioid injection. Available narcotic antagonists include cyclazocine, naloxone, naltrexone, and buprenorphine. Naltrexone, a nearly pure antagonist, seems to be the most promising in initial trials (Resnick et al., 1979), while buprenorphine, a mixed agonist-antagonist, may prove more acceptable to opioid abusers (Jasinski et al., 1978).

Therapeutic communities (e.g., Synanon, Odyssey House, Daytop, Phoenix House) are drug-free, full-time residential programs that attempt to rehabilitate and resocialize the drug addict through the use of a rigidly defined experiential life-style that emphasizes group interaction, peer pressure, and self-government. Treatment in the typical therapeutic community lasts one to two years. It is most effective for the highly motivated individual who can complete the required program (Mirin & Meyer, 1978; Sells, 1979).

Other drug-free outpatient treatment programs provide various resocialization experiences, such as group discussions, assistance with social and vocational problems, and recreational activities. Some are organized along the lines of a daytime therapeutic community (Sells, 1979).

Detoxification programs have the limited goal of withdrawal from the addicting drug during a 7–21 day schedule (see Treatment section on Withdrawal and Withdrawal Deliria).

Outcome studies of long-term treatment and rehabilitation programs for opioid addicts show that methadone maintenance and therapeutic communities are the most successful approaches (Sells, 1979; Simpson, 1981).

305.4x   **Barbiturate or Similarly Acting Sedative or Hypnotic Abuse**
304.1x   **Barbiturate or Similarly Acting Sedative or Hypnotic Dependence**
305.6x   **Cocaine Abuse**

305.7x   Amphetamine or Similarly Acting Sympathomimetic Abuse
304.4x   Amphetamine or Similarly Acting Sympathomimetic
          Dependence
305.9x   Phencyclidine (PCP) or Similarly Acting
          Arylcyclohexylamine Abuse
305.3x   Hallucinogen Abuse
305.2x   Cannabis Abuse
304.3x   Cannabis Dependence

These classes of substances, commonly referred to as "soft" drugs, are discussed together because they share common aspects regarding the treatment of disorders associated with their abuse. These drugs are very often used in combination by multidrug abusers. Detoxification and treatment of psychiatric complications (Organic Brain Syndromes) associated with the use of these substances were discussed elsewhere (see Treatment of Organic Mental Disorders).

Severity of the disorder varies according to the type of substance used. Dependence on sedative-hypnotics is the most serious and most difficult to treat, while cocaine, hallucinogen, and cannabis abuse present a relatively more favorable prognosis. Polydrug abuse with these classes of substances often involves alcohol abuse. Underlying psychopathology is a common problem, especially with the polydrug abuser, and usually involves depression and personality disorders or both. Treatment of the underlying psychiatric disorder is a necessary condition for the long-term rehabilitation of these patients.

Detoxification is a prerequisite in the treatment of these disorders (see respective sections). Following thorough psychiatric evaluation, the patient should be referred for long-term psychiatric treatment. Psychotherapy is the method of choice for most of these patients, although its efficacy has not been established. The major goal of therapy is the establishment of a therapeutic alliance and the use of the therapeutic relationship as a means of treating the underlying psychiatric disorder. Antidepressants and lithium are effective in the treatment of those suffering from affective disorders. Referral to drug-free outpatient treatment programs and utilization of community service support agencies are an important aspect of management. Unfortunately, most patients are not sufficiently motivated to pursue treatment; the majority drop out after the initial evaluation (Anderson et al., 1972). Treatment in a therapeutic community with a rigorously structured resocialization program provides the greatest chance for success, especially for the highly motivated or legally incarcerated individual (Sells, 1979). Generally, the longer a person stays in treatment the more favorable the outcome (Simpson, 1981).

305.1x   Tobacco Dependence

In contrast to other substance use disorders, tobacco dependence is not associated with impairment in social or occupational functioning. There are numerous treatment methods, reporting varying rates of success. Behavioral and psychotherapeutic techniques include aversive conditioning, desensitization, covert desensitization, hypnotherapy, group therapy, supportive therapy, and education therapy. Several educational programs are available for smokers interested in giving up the habit. The best results are seen in programs that combine education with group therapy and support. In spite of reported high rates of success for some programs, the majority of smokers revert to the original habit. The best method is abrupt abstinence when motivation is high (Jarvik et al., 1977). Pharmacological methods using lobeline sulfate (a nicotine agonist), nicotine gum, sedatives, or psychostimulants have not been proven effective (Hunt & Bespalec, 1974; Jaffe & Jarvik, 1978; Jarvik et al., 1977).

305.9x	Other, Mixed, or Unspecified Substance Abuse
304.6x	Other Specified Substance Dependence
304.9x	Unspecified Substance Dependence
304.7x	Dependence on a Combination of Opioid and Other Nonalcoholic Substance
304.8x	Dependence on a Combination of Substances, Excluding Opioids and Alcohol

Other Substance Abuse (305.9x) and Other Specified Substance Dependence (304.6x) refer to substances not classified in any of the previously discussed categories: for instance, abuse of inhalant volatile hydrocarbons (e.g., glue, paint) or amyl nitrate, or dependence on codeine or corticosteroids.

Polydrug abuse (Mixed Substance Abuse, 305.9x) and polydrug dependence involve more than one nonalcoholic substance category. Dependence on a Combination of Opioid and Other Nonalcoholic Substances (304.7x) often involves a combination of heroin and barbiturates. Dependence on a Combination of Substances, Excluding Opioids and Alcohol (304.8x) often involves a combination of amphetamines and barbiturates.

Polydrug abusers are more likely to show significant psychopathology than single substance abusers. Treatment of the concomitant psychiatric disorder is of paramount significance. Detoxification of patients with mixed drug dependence was discussed in the Treatment section on Withdrawal and Withdrawal Deliria.

References

American Psychiatric Association: *Diagnostic and Statistical Manual of Mental Disorders*, 3rd Edition. Washington, D.C.: American Psychiatric Association, 1980.

Anderson, W., O'Malley, J. E., and Lazare, A.: Failure of outpatient treatment of drug abuse: Amphetamines, barbiturates, hallucinogens. *American Journal of Psychiatry*, 182:122–125, 1972.

Aniline, O., Allen, R. E., and Pitts, F. N.: Treatment of PCP intoxication and abuse. In *Syllabus and Scientific Proceedings*. Washington, D.C.: American Psychiatric Association, 1981, p. 31.

Atsmon, A., and Blum, I.: The discovery. In E. Roberts and P. Amacher (Eds.), *Propranolol and Schizophrenia*. New York: Alan R. Liss, 1978, pp. 5–38.

Ayd, F. J.: Haloperidol: Twenty years' clinical experience. *Journal of Clinical Psychiatry*, 39: 807–814, 1978.

Balis, G. U. (Ed.): Delirium and other states of altered consciousness. *The Practice of Medicine*. Volume 10. Hagerstown, MD: Harper and Row, 1970.

Balis, G. U.: The use of psychotomimetic and related consciousness-altering drugs. In S. Arieti, (Ed.), *American Handbook of Psychiatry*, Vol. 3. New York: Basic Books, 1974, pp. 404–445.

Balis, G. U.: Behavior disorders associated with epilepsy. In G. U. Balis, L. Wurmser, E. McDaniel, and R. G. Grenell (Eds.), *Clinical Psychopathology, Psychiatric Foundations of Medicine, Vol. 4*. Boston: Butterworth, 1978, pp. 3–64.

Balis, G. U.: The effects of drugs in episodic dyscontrol disorders. In S. Fielding and R. C. Effland (Eds.), *New Frontiers in Psychotropic Drug Research*. New York: Futura Publishing Co., 1979, pp. 191–240.

Balis, G. U.: Criterion value of atypical drug responses in the diagnosis of atypical psychiatric disorders. *Journal of Nervous and Mental Disease*, 170(12):737–743, 1982.

Ban, T. A.: Vasodilators, stimulants and anabolic agents in the treatment of geropsychiatric patients. In M. A. Lipton, A. DiMascio, and K. F. Killam (Eds.), *Psychopharmacology: A Generation of Progress*. New York: Raven Press, 1978a.

Ban, T. A.: The treatment of depressed geriatric patients. *American Journal of Psychotherapy*, 32:93–104, 1978b.

Berger, P. A., and Tinklenberg, J. R.: Medical management of the drug abuser. In A. M. Freeman, R. L. Sack, and P. L. Berger (Eds.), *Psychiatry For The Primary Care Physician*. Baltimore: Williams and Wilkins, 1979, pp. 359–380.

Bigger, J. T., Kantor, S. J., Glassman, A. H., et al.: Cardiovascular effects of tricyclic antidepressant drugs. In M. A. Lipton, A. DiMascio, and K. F. Killam (Eds.), *Psychopharmacology: A Generation of Progress.* New York: Raven Press, 1978.

Blumenthal, M. D., and Davie, J. W.: Dizziness and falling in elderly psychiatric outpatients. *American Journal of Psychiatry,* 137:203–206, 1980.

Blumer, D.: Temporal lobe epilepsy and its psychiatric significance. In D. Benson and D. Blumer (Eds.), *Psychiatric Aspects of Neurological Disease.* New York: Grune & Stratton, 1975.

Blumer, D.: Treatment of patients with seizure disorders referred because of psychiatric complications. *McLean Hospital Journal,* 53, June 1977.

Brady, J. P., Foulks, E. T., Childress, A. R., and Pertshuk, M.: The Michigan Alcoholism Screening Test as a survey instrument. *Journal of Operational Psychiatry,* 13:27–31, 1982.

Brust, J. C. M.: "Release hallucinosis" as the major symptom of posterior cerebral artery occlusion: A report of two cases. *Annals of Neurology,* 2:432, 1977.

Butler, R. W.: Psychotherapy of old age. In S. Arieti (Ed.), *American Handbook of Psychiatry,* Vol. 5. New York: Basic Books, 1975, pp. 807–828.

Cade, J. F. J.: Massive thiamine dosage in the treatment of acute alcoholic psychosis. *Australia and New Zealand Journal of Psychiatry,* 6:222–230, 1970.

Caine, E. D.: Pseudodementia. *Archives of General Psychiatry,* 38:1359–1364, 1981.

Charney, D. S., Sternberg, D. E., Kleber, H. D. et al.: The clinical use of clonidine in abrupt withdrawal from methadone. *Archives of General Psychiatry,* 38:1273–1277, 1981.

Cole, J. O., and Braconnier, M. A.: Drugs and senile dementia. In J. O. Cole (Ed.), *Psychopharmacology Update.* Lexington, MA: Collamore Press, 1980.

Cummings, J., Benson, D., and LoVerme, S.: Reversible dementias. *Journal of the American Medical Association,* 243:2434–2439, 1980.

Czechowicz, D.: *Detoxification Treatment Manual.* Rockville, MD: National Institute of Drug Abuse, U.S. Dept. of Health, Education, and Welfare, 1978.

Davies, R. K., Tucker, G. J., Harrow, M., et al.: Confusional episodes and antidepressant medication. *American Journal of Psychiatry,* 128:95–99, 1971.

Davis, J. M., and Benvenuto, J. A.: Acute reactions from drug abuse problems. In H. L. P. Resnick and H. L. Ruben (Eds.), *Emergency Psychiatric Care.* Bowie, MD: Charles Press, 1975, pp. 81–101.

Davis, J. M., Sekerke, J., and Janowski, D.: Drug interactions involving drugs of abuse. In National Commission on Marijuana and Drug Use, *Drug Use in America: Problem in Perspective* (Second report of the National Commission on Marijuana and Drug Use). Washington, D.C.: U.S. Government Printing Office, 1973.

Dubovsky, S. L., and Weisberg, M. P.: *Clinical Psychiatry in Primary Care,* 2nd Ed. Baltimore, MD: Williams & Wilkins, 1982, pp. 102–103.

Ellinwood, E. H.: Amphetamines/anorectics. In R. I. DuPont, A. Goldstein, and J. O'Donnell (Eds.), *Handbook of Drug Abuse,* Washington, D.C.: U.S. Government Printing Office, National Institute on Drug Abuse, DHEW, 1979, pp. 221–231.

Falk, W. E., Mahnke, M. W., and Poskanzer, D. C.: Lithium prophylaxis of cortico-tropin-induced psychosis. *Journal of the American Medical Association,* 241:1011–1012, 1979.

Fraser, J. F., Isbell, H., Eisenman, A. J., Wikler, A., and Pescor, F. T.: Chronic barbiturate intoxication: Further studies. *Archives of Internal Medicine,* 94:34–41, 1964.

Freinkel, N., and Arky, R. A.: Effects of alcohol on carbohydrate metabolism in man. *Psychosomatic Medicine,* 28:551–563, 1966.

Gaitz, C. M., Varner, R. V., and Overall, J. E.: Pharmacotherapy for organic brain syndrome in late life. *Archives of General Psychiatry,* 34:839–845, 1977.

Gerard, D. L., and Saenger, G.: *Outpatient Treatment of Alcoholism.* Toronto: University of Toronto Press, 1966.

Gerner, R., Estabrook, W., Stever, J., et al.: Treatment of geriatric depression with trazodone, imipramine, and placebo: A double-blind study. *Journal of Clinical Psychiatry,* 41:216–220, 1980.

Gershon, S., Neubauer, H., and Sundland, D. M.: Interaction between some anticholinergic agents and phenothiazines. *Clinical Pharmacology and Therapeutics,* 6:749–776, 1965.

Glassman, A. H., Giardina, E. V., Perel, J. M., et al.: Clinical characteristics of imipramine-induced orthostatic hypotension. *Lancet*, 1:468–472, 1979.

Gold, M. S., Pottash, A. C., and Extein, I.: Hypothyroidism and depression. *Journal of the American Medical Association*, 245:1919–1922, 1981.

Gold, M. S., Pottash, A. C., Sweeney, D. R., et al.: Opiate withdrawal using clonidine. *Journal of the American Medical Association*, 243:343–346, 1980.

Goldfrank, L., and Meliek, M.: Locoweed and other anticholinergics. *Hospital Physician*, 8: 13–39, 1979.

Goldstein, A., and Judson, B. A.: Efficacy and side effects of three widely different methadone doses. In *Proceedings of the Fifth National Conference on Methadone Treatment*. New York: National Association for the Prevention of Addiction to Narcotics, 1973.

Goodwin, E. W.: Substance induced and substance use disorders: Alcohol. In J. H. Greist, J. W. Jefferson, and R. L. Spitzer (Eds.), *Treatment of Mental Disorders*. New York: Oxford University Press, 1982, pp. 44–61.

Granacher, R. P., Baldessarini, R. J., and Messner, E.: Physostigmine treatment of delirium induced by anticholinergics. *American Family Physician*, 13:99–103, 1976.

Greden, J. F.: Caffeine and tobacco dependence. In H. I. Kaplan, A. M. Freedman, and B. J. Sadock (Eds.), *Comprehensive Textbook of Psychiatry*. Vol. 2. Baltimore, MD: Williams and Wilkins, 1980, pp. 1645–1652.

Green, A. I., Meyer, R. E., and Shader, R. I.: Heroin and methadone abuse: Acute and chronic management. In R. I. Shader (Ed.), *Manual of Psychiatric Therapeutics: Practical Psychopharmacology and Psychiatry*. Boston: Little, Brown, 1975.

Greenblatt, D. J., and Shader, R. I.: Treatment of the alcoholic withdrawal syndrome. In R. I. Shader (Ed.), *Manual of Psychiatric Therapeutics*. Boston: Little, Brown, 1975.

Hamilton, L. D.: Aged brain and the phenothiazines. *Geriatrics*, 21:131–138, 1966.

Heizer, J. R., and Wilbert, D. E.: Reversal of delirium induced by tricyclic antidepressant drugs with physostigmine. *American Journal of Psychiatry*, 131:1275–1276, 1974.

Hollister, L. E., Montzenbecker, R. P., and Degans, R. O.: Withdrawal reactions from chlordiazepoxide. *Psychopharmacologia*, 2:63–68, 1966.

Hrdina, P. D., Rovei, V., Henry, J. F., et al.: Comparison of single-dose pharmacokinetics of imipramine and maprotiline in the elderly. *Psychopharmacology*, 70:29–34, 1980.

Hunt, W. A., and Bespalec, D. A.: An evaluation of current methods of modifying smoking behavior. *Journal of Clinical Psychology*, 30:431–438, 1974.

Ifabumuyi, O. L., and Jeffries, J. J.: Treatment of drug-induced psychosis with diphenylhydantoin. *Canadian Psychiatric Association Journal*, 21:565–569, 1976.

Jaffe, J. H., and Jarvik, M. E.: Tobacco use and tobacco use disorder. In M. A. Lipton, A. DiMascio, and K. F. Killam (Eds.), *Psychopharmacology: A Generation of Progress*. New York: Raven Press, 1978, pp. 1665–1676.

Jarvik, M. E., Cullen, J. W., Gritz, E. R., Vogt, T. M., and West, L. J.: *Research on Smoking Behavior*. National Institute on Drug Abuse, Research Monograph Series #17, DHEW. Washington, D.C.: U.S. Government Printing Office, 1977.

Jasinski, D. R., Pevnick, J. S., and Griffith, J. D.: Human pharmacology and abuse potential of the analgesic buprenorphine. *Archives of General Psychiatry*, 35:501–516, 1978.

Khantziam, E. J., and McKenna, G. J.: Acute toxic and withdrawal reaction associated with drug use and abuse. *Annals of Internal Medicine*, 90:361–372, 1979.

Kissin, B., Lowinson, J. H., and Millman, R. B.: Recent Developments in Chemotherapy of Narcotic Addiction. *Annals of the New York Academy of Sciences*, Vol. 311, 1978.

Krauthammer, C., and Klerman, G. L.: Secondary mania: Manic syndromes associated with antecedent physical illness or drugs. *Archives of General Psychiatry*, 35: 1333, 1978.

Kuhn, R.: The psychotropic effect of carbamazepine in non-epileptic adults, with particular reference to the drug's possible mechanism of action. In W. Birkmayer (Ed.), *Epileptic Seizures-Behavior-Pain*. Baltimore, MD: University Park Press, 1976, pp. 268–271.

Lehman, H. E., and Ban, T. A.: Central nervous stimulants and anabolic substances in geropsychiatric therapy. In S. Gershon and A. Raskin (Eds.), *Aging, Vol. 2: Genesis and Treatment of Psychologic Disorders in the Elderly*. New York: Raven Press, 1975.

Leigh, D.: Psychiatric aspects of head injury. *Psychiatry Digest,* 40:21, 1979.

Lewis, D. C., and Senay, E. C.: *Treatment of Drug and Alcohol Abuse.* Medical Monograph Series, Vol. II, No. 2, Career Teacher Center, State University of New York Downstate Medical Center, New York, 1981.

Lezak, M. D.: Living with the characterologically altered brain injured patient. *Journal of Clinical Psychiatry,* 39:592–598, 1978.

Ling, W., and Blaine, J. D.: The Use of LAAM in Treatment. In R. I. DuPont, A. Goldstein, and J. O'Donnell (Eds.), *Handbook on Drug Abuse.* Washington, D.C.: U.S. Government Printing Office, National Institute on Drug Abuse, DHEW, 1979, pp. 87–96.

Lipowski, Z. J.: Organic brain syndromes: Overview and classification. In D. F. Benson and D. Blumer (Eds.), *Psychiatric Aspects of Neurologic Disease.* New York: Grune and Stratton, 1975, pp. 11–35.

Lipowski, Z. J.: Organic mental disorders: Introduction and review of syndromes. In H. I. Kaplan, A. M. Freedman, and B. J. Sadock (Eds.), *Comprehensive Textbook of Psychiatry.* Baltimore, MD: Williams and Wilkins, 1980 (a), pp. 1359–1392.

Lipowski, Z. J.: *Delirium. Acute Brain Failure in Man.* Springfield IL: Charles C Thomas, 1980 (b).

Marini, J. L., and Sheard, M. H.: Antiaggressive effect of lithium in man. *Acta Psychiatrica Scandinavica,* 55:269–286, 1977.

McAllister, T. W., and Price, T. R. P.: Severe depressive pseudodementia with and without dementia. *American Journal of Psychiatry,* 139:626–629, 1982.

Mendelson, J. H.: Biologic concomitants of alcoholism. *New England Journal of Medicine,* 283: 24–32, 1970.

Mirin, S. M., and Meyer, R. E.: Treatment of substance abusers. In W. G. Clark and J. Del Guidice (Eds.), *Principles of Psychopharmacology.* New York: Academic Press, 1978, pp. 701–720.

Monroe, R. R.: Anticonvulsants in the treatment of aggression. *Journal of Nervous and Mental Disease,* 1960:119–126, 1975.

Moore, D. P.: Rapid treatment of delirium in critically ill patients. *American Journal of Psychiatry,* 134:1431–1432, 1977.

O'Donnell, J. A.: *Narcotic Addicts in Kentucky.* (U.S. Public Health Service Publication No. 1881). Washington, D.C.: U.S. Government Printing Office, 1969.

Ogata, M., Mendelson, J., and Mello, N.: Electrolytes and osmolarity in alcoholics during experimental intoxication. *Psychosomatic Medicine,* 30:463–488, 1968.

Patten, B. M.: Modality-specific memory disorders in man. *Acta Neurologica Scandinavica,* 48: 69–86, 1972.

Peters, B. H., and Levin, H. S.: Memory enhancement after physostigmine treatment in the amnestic syndrome. *Archives of Neurology,* 34:215–219, 1977.

Peterson, P.: Psychiatric disorders in primary hyperparathyroidism. *Journal of Clinical Endocrinology,* 28:1491–1495, 1968.

Plutzky, M.: Principles of psychiatric management of chronic brain syndrome. *Geriatrics,* 29: 120–127, 1974.

Preskorn, S. H., and Simpson, S.: Tricyclic-antidepressant-induced delirium and plasma drug concentration. *American Journal of Psychiatry,* 139:822–823, 1982.

Puente, R. M.: The use of carbamazepine in the treatment of behavioral disorders in children. In W. Birkmeyer (Ed.), *Epileptic Seizures-Behavior-Pain.* Baltimore, MD: University Park Press, 1976, pp. 243–247.

Reisberg, B.: Office management and treatment of primary degenerative dementia. *Psychiatric Annals,* 12:631–642, 1982.

Reisberg, B., Ferris, S. H., and Gershon, S.: An overview of pharmacologic treatment of cognitive decline in the aged. *American Journal of Psychiatry,* 138:593–600, 1981.

Resnick, R. B., Schuyton-Resnick, E. S., and Washton, A. M.: Treatment of opioid dependence with narcotic antagonists: A review and commentary. In R. I. DuPont, A. Goldstein, and J. O'Donnell (Eds.), *Handbook on Drug Abuse.* Washington, D.C.: U.S. Government Printing Office, National Institute on Drug Abuse, DHEW, 1979, pp. 97–104.

Robinson, D. S.: Age-related factors affecting antidepressant drug metabolism and clinical response. In K. Nancy (Ed.), *Geriatric Psychopharmacology*. New York: Elsevier/North Holland, 1979.

Roose, S., Glassman, A. H., Siris, S., et al.: Comparison of imipramine and nortriptyline induced orthostatic hypotension: A meaningful difference. *Journal of Clinical Psychopharmacology*, 1:316–321, 1981.

Rothstein, E., Cobble, J. C., and Sampson, N.: Chlordiazepoxide: Long-term use in alcoholism. *Annals of the New York Academy of Sciences*, 273:381–384, 1976.

Sakles, C. J., and Balis, G. U.: Acute brain syndromes. In G. U. Balis, L. Wurmser, E. McDaniel, and R. G. Grenell (Eds.), *Clinical Psychopathology, The Psychiatric Foundations of Medicine*, Vol. 4. Boston: Butterworth, 1978, pp. 65–86.

Salzman, C.: Electroconvulsive therapy. In R. I. Shader (Ed.), *Manual of Psychiatric Therapeutics*. Boston: Little, Brown, 1975.

Salzman, C.: Update on geriatric psychopharmacology. *Geriatrics*, 34:87–90, 1979.

Salzman, C.: A primer on geriatric psychopharmacology. *American Journal of Psychiatry*, 139: 67–74, 1982.

Salzman, C., Shader, R. I., and Pearlman, M.: Psychopharmacology and the elderly. In R. I. Shader and A. DiMascio (Eds.), *Psychotropic Drug Side Effects*. Baltimore, MD: Williams & Wilkins, 1970.

Sellers, E. M., and Kalant, H.: Alcohol intoxication and withdrawal. *New England Journal of Medicine*, 294:757–762, 1976.

Sells, S. B.: Treatment effectiveness. In R. I. DuPont, A. Goldstein, and J. O'Donnell (Eds.), *Handbook on Drug Abuse*. Washington, D.C.: U.S. Government Printing Office, National Institute on Drug Abuse, DHEW, 1979, pp. 105–118.

Selzer, M. L.: Alcoholism and alcoholic psychosis. In H. I. Kaplan, A. M. Freedman, and B. J. Sadock (Eds.), *Comprehensive Textbook of Psychiatry, III*. Baltimore, MD: Williams and Wilkins, 1980, pp. 1629–1645.

Selzer, M. L., Vinokur, A., and Von Rooijen, L. A.: A self-administered short Michigan Alcoholism Screening Test (MAST). *Journal of Studies on Alcohol*, 36:117–126, 1975.

Sheard, M. H.: The effect of lithium in the treatment of aggression. *Journal of Nervous and Mental Disease*, 160:108–118, 1975.

Sheard, M. H., Marini, J. L., Bridges, C. K., et al.: The effect of lithium on impulsive aggressive behavior in man. *American Journal of Psychiatry*, 13:1409–1413, 1976.

Simpson, D. D.: Treatment for drug abuse. *Archives of General Psychiatry*, 38:875–880, 1981.

Smith, D. L., and Wesson, D. R.: A new method of treatment of barbiturate dependence. *Journal of the American Medical Association*, 2:294–295, 1970.

Solursh, L. P., and Clement, W. R.: Hallucinogenic drug abuse: Manifestations and management. *Canadian Medical Association Journal*, 98:407–410, 1968.

Stending-Lindberg, G.: Hypomagnesemia in alcohol encephalopathies. *Acta Psychiatrica Scandinavica*, 50:465–480, 1974.

Stern, M.: Office management of organic mental disorders. *Psychiatric Annals*, 12:618–630, 1982.

Storey, P. B.: Brain damage and personality change after subarachnoid hemorrhage. *British Journal of Psychiatry*, 117:129–142, 1970.

Taylor, R. L., Maurer, J. I., and Tinklenberg, J. R.: Management of "bad trips" in an evolving drug scene. In C. P. Rosenbaum, and J. E. Beebe (Eds.), *Psychiatric Treatment*. New York: McGraw-Hill, 1975, pp. 155–160.

The Medical Letter, Vol. 23 (3) (Issue 576), February 6, 1981.

Troupin, A. S.: Carbamazepine in epilepsy. In H. L. Klawans (Ed.), *Clinical Neuropharmacology*, Vol. 3. New York: Raven Press, 1978.

Tunks, E. R., and Dermer, S. W.: Carbamazepine in the dyscontrol syndrome associated with limbic system dysfunction. *Journal of Nervous and Mental Disease*, 164:56–63, 1977.

Tupin, J. P.: Usefulness of lithium for aggressiveness (letter to the Editor). *American Journal of Psychiatry*, 135:1118, 1978.

Victor, M., and Adams, R. D.: The effect of alcohol on the nervous system. In *Proceedings of the Association for Research in Nervous and Mental Disease*. Baltimore, MD: Williams and Wilkins, 1953.

Victor, M., Adams, R. C., and Collins, G. H.: *The Wernicke-Korsakoff Syndrome*. Philadelphia: A. Davis, 1971.

Vohra, J., Burrows, G. D., and Solman, G.: Assessment of cardiovascular side effects of therapeutic doses of tricyclic antidepressant drugs. *Australia and New Zealand Journal of Medicine*, 5:7-11, 1975.

Washton, A. M., and Resnick, R. B.: Clonidine for opiate detoxification: Outpatient clinical trials. *American Journal of Psychiatry*, 137:1121-1122, 1980.

Wells, C. E.: Pseudodementia. *American Journal of Psychiatry*, 136:895-900, 1979.

Westermeyer, J.: *Primer on Chemical Dependence*. Baltimore, MD: Williams and Wilkins, 1976.

Whitfield, C. L.: Outpatient management of the alcoholic patient. *Psychiatric Annals*, 12:447-458, 1982.

Whitlock, F. A., and Evans, L. E. J.: Drugs and depression. *Drugs*, 15:53-71, 1978.

Wulff, M. H.: The barbiturate withdrawal syndrome: A clinical and electroencephalographic study. *Electroencephalographic Clinical Neurophysiology*, Suppl. 14:1-173, 1959.

Yesavage, J. A., Tinklenberg, J. R., Hollister, L. E., et al.: Vasodilators in senile dementia: A review of the literature. *Archives of General Psychiatry*, 36:220-223, 1979.

Section III

by

William H. Reid, M.D., M.P.H.

Chapter 4

Schizophrenic Disorders

With few exceptions, general treatment is similar for each of the first four listed types of schizophrenia (Disorganized, Catatonic, Paranoid, Undifferentiated). There are some differences in presentation, motivation for treatment, acceptance of treatment, adaptation to the treating institution and to the community, and prognosis; however, the principles of psychiatric intervention vary little. In addition, our discussion of the treatment of acute schizophrenic psychosis applies as well to Schizophreniform Disorder (295.40; page 126).

295.1x	Schizophrenic Disorder, Disorganized Type
295.2x	Schizophrenic Disorder, Catatonic Type
295.3x	Schizophrenic Disorder, Paranoid Type
295.9x	Schizophrenic Disorder, Undifferentiated Type

Acute Treatment. After appropriate observation, examination, and the ruling out of contraindications to antipsychotic medication, active pharmacologic and milieu treatment should begin.

The author favors the "rapid neuroleptization schedule" described by a number of clinicians (notably Donlon and colleagues [1980]). This should take place in a relatively quiet, nonthreatening milieu (particularly for agitated and/or paranoid patients). The most commonly used agent is haloperidol, which should be given intramuscularly initially, 5–10 mg every 60 minutes until symptoms improve, sedation intervenes, medical complications arise (e.g., hypotension), or the total dose over 12 hours approaches 100 mg. Most patients will require far less. Thiothixene or loxapine may be used in equiva-

113

lent doses; however, the less potent neuroleptics may result in more patient discomfort, sedation, and potential tissue damage (Menuck and Voineskos, 1981).

Oral rapid neuroleptization has also been used, particularly liquid haloperidol and fluphenazine (Donlon et al., 1980); however, absorption and peak serum concentration are significantly delayed and higher doses than those used I.M. may be necessary. Oral treatment may be far preferable when there is no emergency, and when one wishes to minimize issues of control, invasiveness, and future noncompliance.

At least one report indicates that the amount of medication in rapid I.M. neuroleptization with haloperidol may not be as important as the frequency of injection and the intense treatment milieu (Neborsky et al., 1981). This study found that patients receiving injections of 2 mg improved as rapidly as those receiving 10 mg injections, with no significant differences in side effects.

Acute side effects, particularly extrapyramidal symptoms (EPS), should be treated as they arise. The most frightening of these, fairly common among young male patients and often interfering with future trust and medication compliance, is dystonia, which can be rapidly alleviated with intramuscular antiparkinsonian agents. Less severe effects can often be treated with oral drugs or reassurance. EPS or hypotension may not appear for 24 hours after treatment has begun.

The above acute treatment program should be carried out in a specialized inpatient unit or in an emergency room setting which is designed for the treatment of psychiatric patients. Repeated assessment must be made. This author prefers inpatient treatment. There is a small group of patients who may be well known to the treating physician and who may be experiencing a relapse of psychosis without a need for an inpatient milieu. For some such patients remission of the acute psychotic episode within several hours may be possible, and return to the community advisable. Such rapid discharge from acute care presupposes the presence of family or other adequate follow-up away from the hospital.

An alternative method of acute treatment, particularly useful for patients who require more diagnostic observation, those who have more potential for adverse effects to the medication, or those in institutions in which a more conservative pharmacologic approach is used, involves the starting of antipsychotic medication at considerably lower doses, with increases every several days until improvement occurs. A number of patients who come to the hospital highly agitated will respond well to a structured hospital environment which is different from their community living situation. Such patients may deserve an opportunity to improve without "rapid neuroleptization." As they get better, the dose of medication necessary to stabilize the acute condition may be considerably less than that used in the rapid treatment modalities, and the patient may be more amenable to individual and group psychotherapeutic approaches.

It may be noted that a number of attempts have been made to predict patients' response to general or specific antipsychotic medication (Neborsky et al., 1982; van Kammen et al., 1982; Yesavage et al., 1982). At the present time, none of these is sufficiently established to warrant recommendation.

Brief Hospital Treatment. The inpatient milieu for early or brief hospital treatment of the schizophrenias should include a therapeutic combination of architecture, staffing, programs, social structure, respite and expectations of the patient. Each has a place in the providing of a dynamic inpatient experience which will lead to successful transition either to outpatient care or to extended residential treatment.

Architectural requirements vary with clinical philosophy and with the level of agitation of the usual patient population. Persons treated under court order or involuntary commitment may require a closed unit, although the reasons for locked doors may be more administrative and legal than therapeutic. Modern treatment environments combine patient safety with pleasing design, using durable materials to provide warmth, color, texture, adequate illumination, and communication within the unit. There should be space for gathering together as well as for patient privacy. The need to observe patients—for evaluation or protection—should be tempered to avoid the feeling of "being in a fishbowl." When seclusion is used, it should be near other patients and/or staff, not in an isolated area.

Nursing stations should be highly accessible, not hidden away where they are likely to be used as retreats by some staff. The "glass cage" nursing station should be avoided whenever possible, since it combines the worst aspects of the "goldfish bowl," "us *vs* them," and tempting retreat. Access to other aspects of the treatment program, such as dining facilities, occupational therapy (OT), and recreation should be as open as is feasible. This author prefers to have patients dine and play in a non-regimented fashion (e.g., an ordinary cafeteria), avoiding regressive in-room meal service whenever possible.

Staffing should reflect the number and variety of mental health professionals needed to effect the various tasks of medical, social, and educational treatment; administration; ward maintenance, and the like. It goes without saying that each staff member should be competent in his or her particular field and sensitive to the needs—sometimes for intervention or redirection and sometimes for inobtrusive presence—of the patient with acutely disturbed thought process. Staff sex and cultural background may be relevant for some treatment issues. Support for staff from the administrative and medical hierarchies is important, and can be expressed through mutual respect, professional use of a staff member's expertise, and opportunity for further education and training. Care should be taken to recognize and deal with those rare staff members who are exploiting, hostile, or otherwise unprofessional in the care of their patients. By the same token, recognition of the toll taken on staff by continuous work with difficult, sometimes frustrating patients is important.

The active inpatient milieu should contain some level of programming during most of the patient's waking hours. At times this may be somewhat intense, such as therapeutically-oriented ward meetings or other highly organized activity. At other times organization is evident but the structure less pronounced, as in individualized activity therapy or at mealtime. Even completely "free" periods should have some semblance of structure, perhaps by virtue of their scheduled nature or the availability of optional alternatives. Programming should be neither intrusive nor overstimulating; rather, it should provide an atmosphere of security and consistency, in which the patient's world is predictable in a caring sort of way.

The brief treatment unit must provide a socializing and therapeutic environment which is dynamic, rather than static. The patient is not expected to merely remain here while the medication does its work or the psychosis remits of its own accord. In the best of circumstances, the patient is engaged in a multimodal environment through which he or she moves and emerges as an outpatient (or extended-stay residential patient) with the best possible opportunity for further and continued improvement.

With this in mind, discharge planning should begin early, within the first few days of hospitalization. Evaluation of the pre-hospital environment and the expected post-hospital environment is used to prepare the patient to leave, and to prepare those in the community to receive and work with him. Brief psychotherapy in a "normalizing" environment, family visits and meetings, practical counseling, and realistic transition plans are the order here. Extensive or exploratory psychotherapy should not be started unless it is to be continued after the patient leaves the acute care unit. Relationships formed with staff and other patients, while important, should be gently pursued as relationships which must soon be broken. Encouragement for reintegration into the family and/or community is reality which must be faced, no matter how forbidding or non-therapeutic the outside world may seem.

Finally, transition to outpatient care should be done with meticulous attention to detail. The patient and others must clearly understand all aspects of follow-up. Whenever possible the outpatient therapist or a representative of the future physician or clinic should begin contact before actual discharge from the hospital.

A traditional aspect of hospital which is often overlooked in descriptions of clinical milieux is that of respite. A significant component of the patient's psychotic symptoms may be related to special stresses, either from his/her environment or from within him/herself. The hospital should provide a protective setting wherein a process of reorganization and healing can occur. The *giving* of something, perhaps food, is often quieting and reassuring. Even the patient who appears belligerent or controlling may be extremely vulnerable; the "difficult" patient is also one who is ill.

By the same token, the dynamic inpatient milieu has certain expectations of even the most disorganized schizophrenic patient. At the least, he or she is expected to behave within broad human guidelines, dressing rather than remaining naked, refraining from striking others, and the like. These are not always within the control of the most acutely disturbed patient; however, denying the patient basic expectations and responsibilities over long periods of time because of his "illness" can come dangerously close to usurping many of his human rights and communicating one's expectation that he will remain sick. This therapeutic posture should not imply foolhardiness, such as endangering the safety of others while expecting an agitated patient to contain himself. Rather, it implies that the patient is a legitimate part of the ward environment, with its reassuring consistency and rules. His responsibilities, insofar as possible, are those of an adult. He is not treated as a child nor patronized, although he and other patients and staff will be protected. He is expected to participate in and be responsible for his care to whatever extent feasible.

Psychopharmacology in early and brief hospitalization. There is no question that the use of antipsychotic medication alleviates or attenuates symptoms in most schizophrenic patients, and significantly shortens hospital stay. In addition, adequate drug treatment in the hospital increases chances of successful outpatient remission and adequate social adjustment (May, Van Putten, et al., 1981). The choice of antipsychotic medication is of less importance than proper, consistent administration and appropriate monitoring for response and side effects. One may wish to have the patient recommend a medication which he or she feels has been most helpful in the past. At this writing, drugs of choice may come from the phenothiazines, butyrophenones, or thioxanthenes. The author often prefers high potency drugs such as fluphenazine, haloperidol, or thiothixene. Some newer antipsychotic preparations are available (e.g., molindone); however, these are generally poor choices for initial treatment except in cases of known previous response to the medication, intolerance for the more established neuroleptics, or particular need for the special side effects profiles of the newer drugs.

Unless side effects are poorly tolerated, the drug which was initially used to control the acute psychosis (if emergency treatment as described at the beginning of this section has taken place) may be continued for intermediate treatment. Initial dosage levels can often be reduced up to 50% once the patient has been stabilized and remission is apparently maximal. Oral administration is preferred for most patients, particularly those with paranoid schizophrenia. Surreptitious administration (e.g., in juice without informing the patient) usually leads to more problems than solutions. Depot preparations such as fluphenazine decanoate should be used with caution at this stage of treatment, since their long-lasting effects are not reversed as easily as those of other injectables, tablets or liquid. The convenience of the depot preparation may not outweigh the disadvantages of invasiveness and infantilization.

Virtually all of the common antipsychotics can be given in once-daily dosage for most patients. Divided doses may alleviate some side effects, such as late evening akathisia. This author does not use any of the fixed-dose drug combinations now marketed in the U.S. (e.g., antipsychotic plus antidepressant), preferring to use multiple medications only when necessary and titrate dosages individually.

It should be remembered that response to most antipsychotics, other than in the rapid neuroleptization protocol mentioned earlier, peaks only after several weeks. The general rule of "give enough, long enough" applies, and can prevent the confusion of frequent medication changes. As mentioned above, therapeutic response is not consistently predicted with "challenge doses" or other methods. Monitoring of serum level of antipsychotics and active metabolites should be used only to verify patient compliance; serum levels are not well correlated with clinical response.

Side effects and adverse effects of antipsychotic medications must be understood by the clinician before they are prescribed, and the ward staff should be trained in the recognition of these and signs of toxicity. Most common side effects can be controlled by titrating the dosage of the drug and/or, in the case of EPS, by antiparkinsonian medication. The addition of this or any other medication adds to clinical considerations in a number of ways, including potential (e.g., anticholinergic) side effects, drug-drug interactions, and alteration of clinical response to the antipsychotic.

Tardive dyskinesia is a serious adverse effect, so far as is currently known, of all antipsychotic medications (with the possible exception of molindone). It may be worsened by common accompanying drugs such as anticholinergic antiparkinsonian preparations. Although it rarely appears during early stages of treatment, the clinician must be familiar with its symptoms and characteristics, since most patients diagnosed "schizophrenic" will have extensive experience with these drugs over the course of their lifetimes.

As in the case for all other psychotropic medications, antipsychotic drugs should not be given in a therapeutic vacuum. The appropriate inpatient milieu has been briefly outlined. In addition, the patient should understand the characteristics of his or her medication, its uses, its drawbacks, and its important place in the overall treatment plan. The single most common reason for rehospitalization of discharged schizophrenic patients is failure to continue medication. The patient who has an understanding of his or her drug treatment and support from the psychiatrist and significant others is more likely to feel he or she is an active participant. This in turn may provide less need to act out using the medication, less fear of its effects, and more understanding of the medication's role in his/her rehabilitation.

Electroconvulsive therapy (ECT). In some studies, ECT has been found useful for several types of acute schizophrenic episodes. Most clinicians feel, however, that pharmacologic treatment is preferable at all stages, with possible exceptions for those patients who have severe affective components, intractable withdrawal, or "malignant catatonia." Even for the treatment-refractory patient, it is probably just as effective to first consider higher doses of the more potent antipsychotic medications (e.g., loxapine up to 300 mg per day) (Lehmann et al., 1981). The very-high-dose approach is most appropriate for young patients, in good physical condition, with relatively short duration of symptoms and some evidence of drug response.

Other treatment. There are a number of other treatment modalities, primarily pharmacologic, which have been used in the past, or might be tried in treatment-refractory patients. Propranolol, while not effective alone, may increase available levels of antipsychotic medication when given with, for example, the phenothiazines (Peet et al., 1981). Work with endorphins and related drugs is still quite experimental (Verhoeven et al., 1982). The use of megavitamins and special diets (e.g., the gluten-free diet [Osborne et al., 1982]) have apparently little or no effect for schizophrenic patients. Hemodialysis has been similarly disappointing in carefully controlled studies (Fogelson et al., 1980). Leukotomy in various forms is rarely used today; however, at least one long-term follow up study suggests that carefully controlled psychosurgery may have been effective in some patients and probably led to less morbidity than is commonly assumed (Benson et al., 1981). Finally, naloxone has been postulated to be useful in the treatment of schizophrenic patients; however, recent studies indicate that it is ineffective when prescribed alone (Pickard Vartanian et al., 1982).

Extended Treatment, Maintenance Treatment. As noted above, the quality of the patient's transition from acute care to maintenance treatment has considerable bearing on adaptation and prognosis. While some characteristics of prognosis are almost certainly determined by characteristics of the schizophrenic illness, length and quality of remissions are favorably affected first by the continuing of medication in adequate doses, and next by the establishment of consistent clinical follow-up.

Medication. Antipsychotic medication does not cure schizophrenia, it suppresses symptoms. For patients whose diagnosis is Brief Reactive Psychosis (298.80), and who thus have specific stressors and time-limited psychoses, medication can be tapered and discontinued. For those with Schizophreniform Disorder (295.40) the possibility of schizophrenia is high; drugs should be discontinued only with caution. The diagnosis of schizophrenia and the prescribing of antipsychotic medications for long periods involve such serious decisions for the clinician that tapering and discontinuing the medication should be carefully attempted for patients who do not meet all of the DSM-III criteria.

Decrease of medication to maintenance levels is recommended, in order to decrease side effects and minimize the total dose of neuroleptic received over the years during which the patient is likely to require such treatment. It is important to wait until the patient's social situation has stabilized (e.g., return to his/her family, establishment of community mental health center visits, etc.) before changing the prescription markedly. Once this transition is complete, most patients can be maintained on as little as half or less of their acute treatment doses.

Depot-injected medications usually have few advantages over oral preparations. In spite of the assumption that patient compliance is increased, careful studies indicate that groups of patients receiving fluphenazine decanoate differ little from those taking oral fluphenazine at the same effective dose. Oral pimozide has a long plasma half-life and is effective when given less than once a day (McCreadie et al., 1982); however, this preparation is not completely accepted as safe and is not available in the United States.

Tardive dyskinesia. In a number of patients, symptoms of tardive dyskinesia will appear after several years of neuroleptic medication. In others the symptoms may appear only when antipsychotic drugs are discontinued, and may be confused with the more benign "withdrawal-emergent-dyskinesia." In spite of a number of studies of potential treatments for this condition, there is at present no approach which is accepted as effective. Increasing the antipsychotic will attenuate or stop tardive dyskinesia in most cases; however, it is clear that this effect is only masking a continuing pathophysiological process which will in the long run be accelerated by the additional drug. Some studies have suggested careful tapering of antipsychotics to allow (in theory) dopamine receptors to become less hypersensitive; however, other work indicates that this does not always protect patients against exacerbation of dyskinetic symptoms. Branchy et al. (1981) report that if one does choose to mask the dyskinesia with a neuroleptic, approximately one-eighth of the initial dose has a masking effect almost equal to that of the original dose.

"Drug holidays" which used to be recommended are now felt to have little or no specific effect on the development of tardive dyskinesia; it appears more logical to establish the lowest effective dose and provide a steady supply of medication.

For most patients and clinicians, the prospect of tardive dyskinesia is extremely upsetting. It is accepted, however, that the benefits of appropriate neuroleptic treatment for chronic schizophrenic patients generally outweigh the risks of developing a serious movement disorder. This is especially true when one considers the tremendous morbidity of the schizophrenic illness, the increasing accuracy of our diagnoses of that condition, the probability that medications will be found in the future which either do not induce tardive dyskinesia or can be used to treat it effectively, and the fact that the dyskinesias almost always develop slowly and are often not permanent in early stages, allowing time for treatment decisions when early neurological symptoms first appear (mouth movements, increased blinking).

Nonpharmacologic aspects of maintenance treatment. These include contact with continuing mental health care; support from the patient's family or others nearby; and a local social network which can assist in the provision of housing, income, social contacts, educational and vocational oppportunity, and general medical care. If one assumes that most of the disabled, chronically mentally ill in community settings are schizophrenic, then available data indicate that some 75% lead less than adequate socially adjusted lives (Talbott, 1982). Talbott feels that no more than 25% of these patients get adequate aftercare (in addition to medication). He reports that housing is the most critical need for these patients, and also reminds us that the incidence of medical illness in this population is roughly three times that of the general population. Continuity of care with attention to practical programs of behavioral modification, learning, social skills, and the like are extremely important. Some studies indicate that in the most active such programs rehospitalization rates may be only about 20% of the rates seen with ordinary "medication-oriented" aftercare programs.

Return to the community is not appropriate for all chronic schizophrenic patients. Some maintenance treatment programs must take place in residential settings such as mental hospitals or nursing homes. These institutions should be equipped to provide for most or all of the needs mentioned with community care in the above paragraph. That is, adequate psychiatric and other medical care should be provided along with appropriate housing, educational and vocational opportunity, social skills training, and recreation. In chronic-care institutions the concept of milieu or community should be at its best. Nursing-home-like institutions tend to be inadequate substitutes for specialized psychiatric care, but may be necessary in many locales.

There are a handful of hospitals in which long-term care is also considered acute treatment. In such settings, many of the characteristics of brief and early hospitalization mentioned above do not apply. The patient, while usually receiving appropriate pharmacological treatment, becomes involved in an intensive attempt at either bolstering needed defenses or actually restructuring portions of the psyche. These approaches are generally psychoanalytically oriented, and require a great investment of energy, time, and money on the part of both patient and clinical staff. Results, for selected patients, are often better than those expected for similar patients who receive brief hospitalization and either community follow-up or ordinary institutional care. The expertise and resources necessary to work in this way are unavailable to most patients and may not be appropriate for many, provided good brief hospitalization and adequate follow-up are available.

A final long-term treatment modality, which should be mentioned but which is usually unavailable and not completely proved, is the community residential facility which accepts patients and encourages them to view their psychotic episodes as useful life events or learning experiences. Such programs, sometimes supported by psychiatrists, appear to work well for a small subset of patients, perhaps those who would have done well in any event. The patient enters an extremely accepting, home-like environment in which he or she is supported and encouraged to experience his symptoms without anxiety, as a sort of phase of his life.

Psychotherapy of schizophrenia. There are a number of psychotherapists and psychoanalysts who treat subacute schizophrenic illness with psychotherapy (with or without medication). A number of principles of psychotherapy of schizophrenia have been outlined by Arieti (1980). He notes that:

1) Therapists should attempt to cause little or no anxiety early in treatment, and should try to diminish anxiety which is already present;
2) the therapist should not wish merely to return the patient to his or her premorbid condition;
3) the therapist must be able to provide and tolerate a delicate balance within the patient, sometimes for several years, before independence from therapy is achieved; and
4) the treatment must be seen as a way in which the patient proceeds toward gradual acceptance of the self.

Arieti points out that at least the first two of these are quite different from psychotherapy of the healthier or neurotic patient. Such a treatment approach is an arduous task for all concerned, and should not be attempted by clinicians without either experience or supervision in this specialized area of psychotherapy.

The presence of a family into which the patient can be reintegrated is important, and many therapists emphasize the family as a major part of restoration of the patient. Although the therapist may recognize serious pathology in the family, which may have victimized or scapegoated the patient, focusing intensely on these problems may interfere with future reintegration.

Group psychotherapy with schizophrenics is much more practical and oriented toward support, developing social skills, and beginning or sustaining relationships rather than toward facilitation of insight (Mosher & Keith, 1979). These are consistent with evidence for the usefulness of practical social support systems and supportive extended family networks.

295.6x   Schizophrenia, Residual Type

Treatment of residual schizophrenia, in which few or no prominent psychotic symptoms are present, follows essentially the same principles as maintenance treatment of any of the other forms of schizoprenia which have improved beyond the acute stage of the illness.

Chapter 5

Paranoid Disorders

297.10   Paranoia
298.30   Acute Paranoid Disorder

Acute Treatment. Acute psychotic presentation of Paranoid Disorder, differentiated from schizophreniform illness or masked depression, is unusual. Treatment of the early stages may be attempted with antipsychotic medication; however, the rapid response seen in schizophreniform psychoses is unlikely for these patients. If the presentation is such that others appear to be in danger (e.g., the patient seems about to take action based upon delusions of persecution or jealousy), then physical management such as hospitalization may be indicated. For those patients who have evidenced dangerousness, a security facility or referral to a law enforcement agency may be the best course.

It should be noted that a number of physical and environmental influences may precipitate symptoms of a paranoid disorder. Understanding and alleviation of, for example, a problem of deafness in an elderly patient may lead to improvement. If paranoia is seen in persons who have recently immigrated from a distant culture, environmental changes (even return to the home country) may be quite helpful. Similarly, changes in environment for demented patients may precipitate paranoid symptoms which may, in turn, respond to reorientation and familiar objects.

Chronic Treatment; Longer Duration of Symptoms. The longer the symptoms have been present, in general, the more refractory they are to simple treatments such as explanation, education, or medication. Some of the culturally induced syndromes, which may take several months to become clinically apparent, may still respond to relocation. If the patient is motivated for treatment and/or the condition mandates some sort of management, antipsychotic medication should be tried with the expectation that it may be poorly tolerated and compliance may be low. Removal of environmental stressors may be helpful; however, individuals and families should not be advised to change life-styles radically (e.g., quit one's job or move to the country) without careful consideration. Psychotherapy tends not to be sought but may be helpful for family members. Other biological therapies such as ECT have not been adequately explored for this condition.

297.30 Shared Paranoid Disorder
In Shared Paranoid Disorder or folie à deux, many clinicians recommend separation of the persons involved, particularly if one of them appears to be a "victim" of the other's pathology (e.g., a child of a psychotic parent). Hospitalization should be considered, in order to provide a supportive environment in which the patient's loss can be resolved and more productive defenses strengthed. Medication may be necessary either for psychosis or for affective symptoms which may develop. Confrontation may be helpful for the "submissive" member of the pair, but should be approached within the complete therapeutic context, not offered by itself.

297.90 Atypical Paranoid Disorder
Other presentations of paranoia which do not meet criteria for organic syndromes, schizophrenias, schizophreniform disorders, paranoid personality disorder, or the above syndromes should be managed according to the clinician's experience, based upon symptoms, underlying psychopathology and motivation for treatment.

Chapter 6

Psychotic Disorders
Not Elsewhere Classified

295.40 Schizophreniform Disorder
Since this disorder meets all criteria for schizophrenia except that of symptom duration, treatment of the acute, early, and maintenance stages are essentially as described in the section on Schizophrenic Disorders (Chapter 4). Two exceptions might be considered:

1) Since the diagnosis of schizophrenia is not clear, although it may be made later, the clinician should feel more free to cautiously decrease maintenance medication and attempt to discontinue drugs in those patients whose symptoms are in good remission. Thus the concept of "indefinite" treatment (drug and otherwise) should not be applied for patients with only the schizophreniform diagnosis.
2) The diagnostic label of "schizophrenia" should be avoided in these patients' records, since it implies a chronic illness with need for potentially toxic medication. The patient should be closely evaluated for symptoms which appear to be those of thought disorder (e.g., schizophrenia) but are in reality related to administration of antipsychotic medication.

298.80 Brief Reactive Psychosis
In the best of clinical settings, the individual who presents acute psychosis without medical signs should be observed for up to several days without drug

treatment. This is particularly useful in patients whose psychotic symptoms appear to have been precipitated by a clear environmental or psychosocial stress (i.e., those who are likely to fit the diagnosis of Brief Reactive Psychosis). For these patients, a supportive, structured environment in which reorganization can occur is likely to lead to rapid attenuation of the psychotic symptoms. Antipsychotic medication, particularly the more potent neuroleptics such as haloperidol, may hasten the disappearance of frank psychosis, even in low doses; however, as with Schizophreniform Disorder, one should be certain that any residual symptoms seen are not the result of the medication itself.

More complete recovery, after the acute psychosis has abated, may take considerable time. Treatment may continue on an open psychiatric unit, although outpatient psychotherapy which focuses on support and reorganization is probably just as effective and likely to lead to fewer future problems. Psychiatric contact, generally without medication, should continue as long as necessary and may involve treatment of conditions described elsewhere in this volume (e.g., Anxiety Disorders).

295.70   Schizoaffective Disorder

Because of the variety of definitions for Schizoaffective Disorder, no specific treatment is recommended. Most authors suggest that primary attention be given to the clinical form taken by the disorder; that is, if the patient seems clinically to suffer more from a thought disorder, then treatments similar to those recommended for the Schizophrenic Disorders should be one's first choice. Conversely, if the symptoms of thought disorder seem secondary to marked affective characteristics such as depression, hypomania, or mood swings, then either antidepressant regimens or lithium should be considered (see Affective Disorders, Chapter 7).

Patients with clear symptoms of both schizophreniform and affective illness often do best with a combination of medications, aimed at treatment of both the apparent thought disorder and the affective symptoms. This author would suggest first treating one or the other. Once the first medication routine has been stabilized, a second may be added if conditions warrant. Fixed-dose preparations should be avoided. As previously stressed, the nonpharmacological components of treatment of both schizophrenic and affective disorders should receive careful consideration in the overall care of the patient.

It may be noted that dysphoria is a common symptom in schizophrenic patients. Drug-induced or post-psychotic depressions are common. Akinetic effects of antipsychotic drugs may be mistaken for depressive withdrawal and psychomotor retardation.

298.90   Atypical Psychosis

These disorders should by and large be treated symptomatically, using the principles outlined for more specific disorders elsewhere in this book. Early treatment should always include careful evaluation for organic, environmental, or other psychosocial causes of the psychosis which might lead one toward or away from certain interventions (such as rapid neuroleptization). When rapid control of acute psychosis is imperative for further evaluation, in order to implement necessary medical treatment or to prevent damage to the patient or others, short-acting barbiturates may be useful without masking important symptoms. Low doses of haloperidol or another potent antipsychotic are safe and may be effective. Neither should be given before evaluating the medical status of the patient.

Chapter 7

Affective Disorders

MAJOR AFFECTIVE DISORDERS

296.4x Bipolar Disorder, Manic
296.5x Bipolar Disorder, Depressed
296.6x Bipolar Disorder, Mixed
Clinical and apparently neurochemical characteristics of the Major Affective Disorders make their treatment more likely than other affective disturbance to require medical intervention including hospitalization, antidepressant or mood-stabilizing medication, convulsive therapy, and/or extensive outpatient follow-up.

296.4x Bipolar Disorder, Manic

Acute Treatment. Acute mania should be considered a medical emergency. It can result in severe physical decompensation or death if not treated promptly.

The first goal of treatment is rapid, safe calming of the patient within a medically supervised setting. Rapid sedation with antipsychotic medication, generally I.M. initially, is a treatment of choice. Some clinicians prefer 5–10 mg of haloperidol I.M. every half hour or hour until control is obtained (see "rapid neuroleptization schedule," page 113). Others prefer the more sedative drugs such as chlorpromazine. In either case, one should expect the patient to require larger amounts than similar patients with other kinds of neuroleptic-responsive psychosis (e.g., schizophreniform psychosis). Monitoring of medical status, particularly blood pressure, is necessary. Medication side effects, most noticeably tremor or dystonia, may appear and should be promptly treated.

An alternative mode of sedation, particularly useful if the diagnosis is in doubt, is administration of short-acting barbiturates. These have the advantage of being sedative without most of the side effects of the neuroleptics, and tend to mask fewer symptoms of psychiatric and medical illness. ECT has been recommended for life-threatening mania but the patient's medical status should be carefully evaluated before proceeding.

Hypomania, Sequelae to Emergency Treatment. Most patients present for treatment at about this level of symptom. If the patient has returned to the office or hospital because of worsening symptoms of an already known illness, one should check for compliance to a previous drug regimen. If the relapse is felt to be related to noncompliance, consider reinstituting the previous treatment in as structured an environment as is felt to be necessary.

If the patient is unfamiliar to the clinician, or has just received emergency treatment for mania, a treatment program designed to control the symptoms and lead to return to the community should be planned at this time. The pharmacologic aspects of this plan include management of manic and hypomanic symptoms with antipsychotic medication (generally orally) and/or the starting of oral lithium carbonate. Lithium is the drug of choice for management of bipolar disorders with manic symptoms; however, stabilization of blood level and alleviation of manic symptoms both require a period of time during which neuroleptics are often necessary.

Before prescribing lithium, the clinician should perform the required pre-lithium medical work-up and be experienced with respect to potential drug interactions, importance of serum level, and recognition of toxicity (which usually affects the gastrointestinal and central nervous systems first).

The milieu in which early treatment takes place is of considerable importance. This author recommends hospitalization, especially for patients who have not taken lithium and whose judgment may interfere with the treatment plan in an unsupervised setting. The hospital milieu should be one in which active or agitated patients are commonly treated, with a staff who are familiar with the special needs of such patients. Locked units, seclusion rooms, or restraints are not usually required provided the staff are familiar with the psychotherapeutic, social, and pharmacologic ways of managing active or agitated patients. The staff should also be familiar with signs of lithium toxicity.

Although these patients may not appear amenable to logic or verbal approaches, a structured setting is important. As the acute symptoms subside, discharge plans should be formulated which address the biological, psychological, and social needs of the patient. Education of the patient and significant others about the special characteristics of bipolar illness and of lithium (particularly toxicity and monitoring) should be provided, with reminders in writing.

Maintenance Treatment. Careful discharge planning and attention to the transition from inpatient to outpatient care are the keys to lasting psychiatric and social post-hospital success. Care should be taken to help the patient with his or her first contact with outpatient treatment, for example providing for visits from the local mental health center while the patient is still in the hospital. At the least, the name and location of the follow-up therapist and a written description of medications and dosages should be in the hands of the patient and/or significant others before he/she leaves the hospital.

Many bipolar patients do not require chronic medication other than lithium to remain in remission. The lithium itself, however, is crucial to preventing relapse. It should not be discontinued without careful supervision; most patients will require treatment for an indefinite period.

Decrease in lithium level, perhaps the most common cause of relapse, may also come from noncompliance by the patient, since return of hypomanic symptoms is rarely perceived as dysphoric. Continued office contact and monitoring of serum lithium levels, as well as the clinician's awareness of special personal or family stressors, may predict potential relapse before it occurs.

A number of factors may affect lithium level in patients in spite of a consistent intake of medication. Any condition which alters electrolyte balance (e.g., dehydration, low salt diet, severe vomiting or diarrhea) alters the serum level and cell membrane transport of the lithium ion. The most common problem is a transient increase in level leading to mild toxicity. Dosage needs may change considerably with age, change in physical condition, pregnancy, or prescription of additional drugs (particularly thiazide diuretics and nonsteroidal anti-inflammatory medications). Serum for lithium level should be obtained at least eight hours after the last dose (12 hours in the case of "slow-release" preparations).

The reader should be familiar with acute side effects of lithium treatment as well as with continuing studies of long-term problems, particularly in the renal and endocrine systems. Renal and thyroid evaluation should be done periodically. For physiologically normal patients lithium therapy is likely to have an excellent risk-to-benefit ratio.

The prognosis is good for most patients, given access to and motivation for appropriate psychiatric care. The prognosis is considerably worsened if there is an absence of a support system for the patient within which signs of relapse can be recognized and treatment compliance encouraged.

Other Treatments. The above regimen is accepted as the modern approach to the treatment of recurrent manic episodes. For those patients who cannot tolerate lithium, chronic antipsychotic medication may be substituted, with a concomitantly poorer prognosis (either because of the treatment or because the illness itself is different). In some patients antipsychotic medication is a necessary adjunct to maintenance lithium treatment. Caution should be used when adding or increasing the antipsychotic medication; both should be discontinued immediately if signs of central nervous system toxicity appear. Electroconvulsive treatment will control acute manic symptoms, but there appears to be little or no advantage in its use except for those patients who do not respond to medication (see beginning of this section).

296.5x   Bipolar Disorder, Depressed

The treatment of acute and subacute depressive episodes, as well as the early treatment of severe depression, is addressed in the section on Major Depression (296.2x, 296.3x; p. 133). The clinical characteristics of depression found in bipolar depressive disorder are essentially those seen in major or "endogenous" depression and can be treated accordingly.

Lithium carbonate is usually not useful in acute depression, even that found in bipolar disorder. Similarly, antipsychotic agents are not ordinarily helpful except for the treatment of specific psychotic symptoms (see Major Depression).

Some authors feel that biological (drug or ECT) treatment of the depression in bipolar, depressed patients (and especially in Bipolar Disorder, Mixed, 296.6x) carries with it the chance of inducing a manic phase. This is not considered a serious risk by most, and concomitant lithium carbonate or neuroleptic treatment should be preventive in those patients who are predisposed to rapid mood swings (Lewis and Winokur, 1982).

Maintenance. Once the depression has been successfully treated, its return may be prevented—or made less likely—in a number of ways. Lithium carbonate will prevent recurrence of depression, once in remission, in most bipolar patients. This is true whether the acute treatment was pharmacologic or with electroconvulsive therapy (Coppen et al., 1981). Continued monitoring for return of symptoms, lithium level, and lithium toxicity is important. As is the case for bipolar, manic patients, the prognosis tends to be good given proper care. Patients with bipolar, depressed illness may be more motivated for treatment because of the marked dysphoria that they experience; on the other hand, their depression may produce apathy and withdrawal from treatment.

As with any depression, suicide remains a risk during the acute phases of the illness as well as during early recovery, when increased activity level and cognitive ability may increase the likelihood of the patient's acting on self-destructive impulses.

296.6x   Bipolar Disorder, Mixed

Acute Treatment. Acute treatment should be consistent with the patient's presentation, either manic (or hypomanic) or severely depressed. Occasionally patients will refer themselves when between mood swings, this being a period of better judgment and some ability to reflect upon the damage done by their symptoms. In such cases, lithium carbonate treatment should be begun at once. Although the patient's apparently stable condition makes it tempting to begin treatment outside the hospital, the author prefers an inpatient evaluation, pre-lithium work-up, stabilization of the medication, and education of the patient and significant others.

Maintenance. Principles of maintenance are taken from those already discussed for the bipolar, manic and bipolar, depressed patients just discussed. The conditions of follow-up and prognosis are similar.

Treatment of Refractory Patients. The careful addition of neuroleptics to the lithium regimen may be helpful in the overall stabilizing of the patient's mood. Some preliminary work with monoamine oxidase inhibitors indicates that they may augment the stabilizing effects of lithium; however, prophylactic use of the tricyclic antidepressants with lithium may increase the probability of a manic relapse for patients with a history of mania.

MAJOR DEPRESSION
The acute and early treatment of these disorders is identical. Differences appear in long-term maintenance (see below).

296.2x   Major Depression, Single Episode
296.3x   Major Depression, Recurrent

Acute Major Depression. Although not as physically disabling as acute mania, the pain and clouded judgment of acute Major Depression make rapid treatment imperative. Initial goals include recognition and management of suicide potential. Hospitalization (even against the patient's will) may be life-saving, and may be recommended if suicide predictors are present, even if the patient has not volunteered information about a history of suicidal ideation or attempts. The patient should be admitted to a secure (but not necessarily locked) unit staffed by persons who are familiar with the treatment of acute depression and management of the suicidal patient. The acute ward milieu should provide for observation and protection of the patient.

The second goal of acute treatment is early alleviation of the tremendous psychic pain found in severe depression. Although antipsychotic medication may be helpful for some aspects of depressive psychosis, treatment with anti-depressants should begin as soon as possible. When rapid lifting of the depression is deemed necessary to prevent suicide, electroconvulsive therapy (ECT) may be a treatment of choice; most antidepressants take several weeks to attain their maximum effect (although some symptoms, such as sleeplessness, may respond much earlier). Some of the newer antidepressant preparations purport to work more rapidly. Amoxapine can show significant effect within four to seven days; however, some patients develop irritability and dysphoria a few weeks later. Alprazolam apparently has antianxiety and possibly antidepressant effects which may prove beneficial within several days. Neither drug has had extensive clinical use in the U.S. at this writing. There are many other considerations in selecting an antidepressant; some of these are described in the section on Treatment Planning below.

Since all known treatments require at least days, and often weeks, before the depression is significantly lifted, attention to nonbiological components of treatment is quite important. Clinical reassurance and understanding from the physician are important to both the patient and his or her family. A word from the psychiatrist that the situation is far from being as hopeless as the patient feels it is can help before the biological treatments take effect. In addition, the clinician should take a firm and unambivalent position with respect to treatment (particularly hospitalization) recommendations rather than waiting for the patient, who is usually ambivalent and whose judgment is significantly clouded by the depressive illness, to decide upon the best course of action. Within the hospital, initial contacts should reflect support and structure, discouraging withdrawal and encouraging adherence to an active milieu program and treatment regimen.

During this acute phase, psychotherapeutic approaches—which may be quite useful later in treatment—are insufficient in and of themselves.

Treatment planning. Once the diagnosis of Major Depression (or depressive phase of Bipolar Disorder, Depressed) has been made and the appropriate treatment setting decided upon, the next step is the choice of the biological treatment which will be tried first. Using the first-choice treatments described below (i.e., tricyclic antidepressants or ECT), there is a greater than 60% likelihood of significant therapeutic response (over 80% for ECT) within four weeks. The dexamethasone suppression test may predict response.

Given a physically healthy patient, not in extreme danger of suicide, the author prefers to begin treatment with a tricyclic antidepressant. If the patient has had recurrent depressions which have responded well to a particular antidepressant, or if there is a family history of severe depression with good response to a particular antidepressant, then this is the agent which should be tried first. Without this predictive history, the clinician may choose a tricyclic which has primarily noradrenergic action (e.g., desipramine), primarily serotonergic action (e.g., amitriptyline), or elements of both (e.g., imipramine). Biochemical methods of predicting which form of medication will be best for a given patient are still considered experimental; most psychiatrists rely on their clinical experience. If the first drug chosen is ineffective even after adequate dosage levels have been maintained for several weeks, one should switch to a tricyclic of the "opposite" reuptake inhibition type (e.g., from desipramine to amitriptyline), with a fair expectation that the change in medication will bring a good response within 10 days to three weeks.

It should be noted that clinical response is not well correlated with circulating plasma level of tricyclic and active metabolites. One may wish to check plasma levels to assess compliance or as a broad measure of whether one is prescribing appropriate doses of medication; however, such measures are not adequate predictors of response itself.

Another means of choosing the first tricyclic, all other things being equal, has to do with the side effects profile. Amitriptyline, for example, is fairly sedative and has significant anticholinergic side effects. While this may quiet the patient, it probably does not have a "specific" effect on agitated patients. Doxepin is said to be less cardiotoxic; however, this is insufficiently established and there appears no particular reason to choose doxepine initially. For patients with significantly compromised cardiac or cardiovascular systems, some of the nontricyclic antidepressants (e.g., maprotiline) may be a first choice; however, in most patients none of the tricyclics will interfere with cardiac or cardiovascular status. Trazodone and nomofensine have almost no anticholinergic side effects. Trazodone is quite sedative; amoxapine and nomofensive are not. Maprotiline has mild-to-moderate sedative and anticholinergic properties.

If the patient does not respond to the first or perhaps the first two choices of antidepressant, then ECT should be considered. Many clinicians would consider it earlier (particularly for the patient with significant cardiac disease), some much later, but the fact remains that with appropriate medical workup ECT is at least as safe as careful prescription of tricyclics—safer in many medically ill patients—and is effective. Ordinary ECT treatment should be unilateral, on the nondominant side, and should be given for several sessions beyond remission of the depressive symptoms. Stopping the treatments as soon as remission occurs is associated with a higher incidence of relapse. The total number of treatments is usually between eight and 12, given at a rate of about three per week. ECT may be given in combination with tricyclic or antipsychotic drugs. Clinicians who use ECT should be comfortable with the medical aspects of this treatment modality and, under the best of conditions, should employ consultation by an anesthesiologist.

Rapid onset of action is an important factor in treatment of the suffering, perhaps suicidal patient. Multiple-monitored ECT (MMECT) may offer considerable advantage in this regard, although the procedure is not universally accepted. There is some evidence that time spent in seizures is more related to improvement than is the number of seizures experienced.

For those patients who refuse ECT, those clinicians who do not wish to use it, and those patients who are treated on an outpatient basis, a variety of further choices of medication is available. (This author does not recommend outpatient ECT for most patients.) The order in which one chooses to try these is of less importance than a careful understanding of the principles of prescribing, the characteristics of the drugs, and the dosage levels and durations necessary before response is expected. Some of the newer "third generation" antidepressants should, at this writing, be considered as later choices, although each has significant literature attesting to its efficacy and safety.

A group of medications which has been available for some time, and which is probably underutilized, is the monoamine oxidase inhibitors (MAOI). Provided the patient understands, and can adhere to, dietary precautions involving high-tyramine foods, these are relatively safe and often effective agents. Phenelzine is a good early choice; tranylcypromine is effective in a slightly different group of patients. In addition to the dietary problems, several other side effects are more common, including orthostatic hypotension and insomnia (which can usually be managed by giving the medication before noon). Dosages of up to 60 mg of phenelzine or 40 mg of tranylcypromine per day are usually sufficient.

The combining of tricyclic antidepressants and MAOIs may be useful for some treatment-resistant patients. The author would reserve this practice for those patients for whom other treatments have failed and for whom ECT has either failed or is unavailable. Although there are hazards involved in combining these two groups of medications, they have been exaggerated in the pre-1980 literature. The safest prescribing regimen is to eliminate any antidepressant for at least one week, then begin both medications together, starting with low doses. The dosage range of each medication should probably not be as high as one might reach with a single drug. The clinician should review the literature in this area before prescribing, and should *not* prescribe tricyclics to a patient who is already taking MAOI.

Other drug combinations that have been tried include tricyclics and liothyronine (T-3) (a sometimes useful combination which seems to have few, if any, complications. The liothyronine is usually given in doses of 25–50 micrograms per day.), tricyclics and neuroleptics (clinically popular but unproved in the literature unless psychotic symptoms are present), MAO inhibitors plus l-tryptophan, and antidepressants plus lithium (*International Drug Therapy Newsletter*, 1981a). In Europe, the intravenous use of tricyclic antidepressants is said to result in increased, more rapid response; however, this practice has not been extensively used in the United States.

Hospital milieu. There are several nonpharmacologic treatment approaches which have considerable use, either alone or with biological treatment. The most important of these for the severely depressed patient is the active hospital milieu. Such a milieu should be structured and supportive, and should discourage withdrawal, apathy, and other regression-encouraging situations. An atmosphere of "firm kindness" presses for physical and emotional activity while providing needed support. Staff should be experienced in the treatment of such patients, and should be particularly aware that the passiveness, dependency, and "manipulation" that are often seen arise from the depressive illness and not usually from dependent or antisocial character style.

Careful transition to outpatient status is important, and has been described in the section on Bipolar Disorders. Particular attention should be paid to the loss that the patient experiences upon leaving (or planning to leave) the hospital, and to the potentially overwhelming prospect of going back to a less-than-perfect home or work environment. Participation of the family in treatment, at least at the stage of discharge planning, is important.

Psychotherapy. Various forms of psychotherapy have been attempted as primary treatments for severely depressed patients. Studies with outpatients (in which the depressive illness was mild enough to allow outpatient treatment) indicate that cognitive therapy is useful alone, and can add considerably to the effectiveness of antidepressant medication. Psychodynamically oriented psychotherapy or psychoanalysis has been reported as successful for some patients; however, studies of its efficacy are lacking. In either case (cognitive or psychodynamic) the therapist must be experienced in this form of treatment, and must understand the depressive illness thoroughly. Behavior modification, again by experienced therapists, is useful for decreasing nonproductive thoughts and activities. Those who use it extensively hope that changing behavior will result in a concomitant change in the patient's general depressive outlook.

Follow-Up and Maintenance. Patients who have responded to biological (drug or ECT) treatment for depression require both medication follow-up and continued adjunctive psychotherapy. The length of necessary follow-up varies; however, premature stopping of medication, by physician or patient, is often associated with relapse. A general rule is that the longer the depression has existed, the longer the patient should continue on an antidepressant, with several months being a minimum. Psychotherapy to help with remnants of depression, assist in social and interpersonal relationships, improve reality testing and deal with situational crises is an important part of treatment.

Many patients will require maintenance medication, at levels as much as 50% lower than the initial dosage, for a number of years. Because of the likelihood of adverse effects from chronic administration of these drugs, it is prudent to attempt to discontinue them (by tapering, not abruptly) every six months or so. Many recurrent depressions (e.g., Bipolar Disorder, Depressed) respond to lithium prophylaxis, which generally has fewer side effects and fewer known long-term adverse effects. The dexamethasone suppression test and/or tests of the TRH-TSH axis may predict the patient's future response to discontinuing medication (i.e., a normalizing of the response indicating no need for the medication), but these should not be relied upon until further established in the literature.

Maintenance drugs probably either mask depressive symptoms (in most cases) or actually prevent them (in the case of lithium carbonate). When symptoms are "masked" our current state of knowledge postulates not an eventual cure, but a keeping away of the symptoms until the depressive episode has run its natural course. This does not seem to be the case for intensive cognitive or psychodynamic treatment successes.

Prognosis. Although depression is the most painful common psychiatric illness, and one of the most painful illnesses of all, both the acute and chronic treatment of its symptoms carries an excellent prognosis. The patients who do not improve considerably are often those who stay away from treatment because of apathy, hopelessness, or withdrawal; those whose families keep them from treatment because of ignorance or stigma; or those who, tragically, commit suicide.

OTHER SPECIFIC AFFECTIVE DISORDERS

301.13 Cyclothymic Disorder

If the relatively mild mood swings of cyclothymia are considered an attenuated form of bipolar disorder, then lithium is a logical treatment of choice (except for specifically depressive symptoms). Unfortunately, controlled research with lithium in specifically diagnosed cases of cyclothymia is lacking. A number of authors consider such patients to be suffering more from character pathology (e.g., narcissistic, histrionic, or borderline traits) than from an affective disorder. From this point of view, particularly if the mood swings are responses to small changes in the patient's physical or emotional environment, psychotherapy or environmental manipulation may be more helpful than medication. Traditional antidepressants (tricyclic or MAOI) or antipsychotic medications are generally not useful.

300.40 Dysthymic Disorder (or Depressive Neurosis)

Acute Treatment. Although dysthymic patients may present with acute depression and concomitant anxiety, the absence of vegetative signs (and usually negative dexamethasone suppression test) predict that antidepressant medication will be of little use. A few recent studies have found trazadone helpful in moderate-to-severe neurotic depression (Goldberg et al., 1981). Early treatment with ineffective antidepressant drugs, which the patient must often take for several weeks for a definitive trial, may interfere with the implementation of valuable psychotherapeutic techniques. Reassurance that the clinician understands the depth of the patient's pain, assessment of suicidal and other self-destructive potential, and optimism for the future are all useful. Pharmacological intervention should generally be limited to acute symptom relief, such as treatment for severe insomnia.

Ongoing Treatment. For almost all patients treatment can take place on an outpatient basis. Patients who receive psychotherapy of any of several types—notably cognitive, interpersonally-oriented, or behavior therapy with social skills training—tend to have a good prognosis, with or without antidepressant medication (Blackburn et al., 1981; Liberman & Eckman, 1981; Weissman et al., 1981). Analytic and other insight-oriented therapies appear useful for some patients, provided specific neurotic conflict patterns can be elucidated, the patient meets other criteria for this form of treatment, and the clinician is experienced in its use.

No matter what the form of psychotherapy, supportive measures are important. These may range from simple reassurance and education of the patient with respect to the characteristics of his or her illness, to unqualified acceptance of the patient who may at times appear hostile or draining to the therapist, to working with significant others in the patient's life. Successful psychotherapy with the depressed patient usually involves warmth and availability on the part of the psychiatrist, and not the classically "neutral" stance which the patient easily misperceives as uncaring.

ATYPICAL AFFECTIVE DISORDERS

296.70 Atypical Bipolar Disorder

Since this DSM-III category is meant for those patients who appear to have clinically significant mood swings but who do not fit criteria for bipolar disorder or cyclothymia, some clinicians recommend beginning treatment based upon the affective symptoms which are seen. That is, hypomania might be treated with lithium, severe depression with antidepressants (both with appropriate psychotherapeutic and social milieux) and maintenance lithium considered once the mood is stabilized. The patient's symptoms may herald more severe mood swings, which will require the treatments described earlier in this section.

296.82 Atypical Depression

As with Atypical Bipolar Disorder, the clinical picture may suggest appropriate biological or psychotherapeutic antidepressant treatment. Since "atypical" means different things to different observers, no one approach can be recommended. The most common interpretations of "atypical" appear to focus on either "reversed vegetative change" (Davidson et al., 1982), in which sleep, appetite, or libido are increased, or upon symptoms of irritability, phobia, hypochondriasis, and fatigue (Stern et al., 1980). In both presentations, MAO inhibitors are recommended if tricyclic antidepressants fail to show good response. Phenelzine appears to be the best studied in such patients. Many reports indicate poor response to ECT.

Chapter 8

Anxiety Disorders

For most patients, treatment of the anxiety disorders can successfully be aimed at alleviating uncomfortable or disabling symptom(s). For some others, for example many patients with a post-traumatic stress disorder, some in-depth treatment may be required or advisable. For patients whose symptoms stem from identifiable neurotic conflict, whose anxieties or compulsions are readily identified by the patient as having to do with more than the particular symptom which brought him or her to the psychiatrist (e.g., "I'm terrified of going outside the house. It's the same feeling I had when my husband went overseas, and when my father was in the hospital"), whose anxiety has not responded to the symptomatic treatments described below, or whose symptom removal appears to lead to the other complaints, insight-oriented psychotherapy designed to address the underlying psychodynamics is often indicated.

In the following pages a number of specific treatment techniques, ranging from the behavioral to the psychoanalytic, will be mentioned. As is the case with any treatment modality, the clinician should be familiar with both the indications and the technical aspects of a given treatment approach before using it or expecting it to be effective. This is true for the apparently simple modalities as well as for those which obviously require extensive training.

PHOBIC DISORDERS (OR PHOBIC NEUROSES)

Behavioral therapy of some sort is the most frequently recommended treatment for most phobias. There is no question that a variety of behavioral approaches will diminish phobic symptoms markedly in most patients (Munby & Johnston, 1980).

300.21   **Agoraphobia with Panic Attacks**
300.22   **Agoraphobia without Panic Attacks**
300.23   **Social Phobia**

The behavioral technique of "exposure" is an effective treatment, both short- and long-term, for agoraphobics and many other phobia patients (Linden, 1981). The use of exposure in fantasy, presenting increasingly anxiety-producing situations as discomfort dissipates at each level, is a form of systematic desensitization. Exposure in vivo also involves gradual adaptation to anxiety-producing objects or situations, but the objects or situations are actually present during the treatment. Flooding, rapid exposure to almost overwhelming volumes of phobic material, also known as implosion, may be used either in fantasy or in vivo.

In the case of an agoraphobic patient, the clinician might have the patient imagine (perhaps in hypnotic trance, but this does not seem to add to the effectiveness of treatment) taking a fearful trip, remaining in the anxiety-producing fantasy as long as possible, then "returning" to the therapist's office. This is repeated a number of times, and the patient is instructed to perform the same exercise as often as possible between sessions. Family members are frequently engaged to assist in the process and monitor the "homework." Written journals and diaries may also be used.

In most patients, panic attacks can be treated at the same time, in the same way. Sometimes attention to the physiologic cues of panic or mounting anxiety helps the patient to recognize and control panic symptoms. The exposure mode of treatment is elegantly described by Marks (1978a & b).

Medications for this and other phobic disorders have been useful in two contexts. First, the minor tranquilizers or anxiolytics are excellent means of treating anxiety symptoms. However, they do not appear to block the actual process of panic attacks (Liebowitz & Klein, 1981). (For further discussion of treatment of Panic Disorder (300.01), see p. 143.) Second, certain of the tricyclic antidepressants have been used in some patients, often in doses well below those used for the Affective Disorders. Imipramine will block some panic attacks and clomipramine (not yet available in the United States) is a promising drug; however, the latter appears of more use in Obsessive Compulsive Disorder (see p. 145) and both have significant side effects. The MAO inhibitors are helpful for some patients. In general, the behavioral treatments, perhaps coupled with appropriate psychotherapy, have the greatest likelihood of effectiveness, and should be tried before medication is prescribed on any chronic basis.

Psychotherapy can be a useful part of the treatment of the anxious or phobic patient. The term "psychotherapy" implies a wide variety of kinds of therapist-patient interaction, overlapping considerably with the behavioral treatments. It is almost impossible to work with a patient in any context without providing considerable interest, support, and understanding. Beyond this, the patient who has given up a symptom may suffer feelings of loss for the symptom itself, for the "equilibrium" of life-style which has existed surrounding the symptom, or both. The opportunity for continuing counseling may be valuable.

Those patients who do not respond to the briefer treatments, and some others mentioned at the beginning of this chapter, often benefit from more in-depth psychodynamic psychotherapy. Andrews and Harvey (1981), in a review of studies of various modes of psychotherapy, found that the typical patient after such treatment was in better condition than 77% of untreated controls evaluated at the same time. The various modes examined included psychodynamic, cognitive, and humanistic, as well as behavioral and social, therapies.

300.29 Simple Phobia
The treatment of Simple Phobia is similar or identical to that described above for the agoraphobias. It should be noted that the term "simple" implies that the phobia has little significant underlying psychopathology present.

ANXIETY STATES (OR ANXIETY NEUROSES)

300.01 Panic Disorder
The primary acute treatment of Panic Disorder, once other problems (particularly organic, including caffeinism) have been ruled out, should be the short-term use of antianxiety medication (especially a benzodiazepine) coupled with brief psychotherapy and reassurance that, although extremely uncomfortable, the disorder does not lead to severe mental illness. A communication to the patient that the symptoms can be managed and very probably transient is helpful. The patient may take the anxiolytic prophylactically or only during acute symptoms. The mere presence of a supply of effective medication in one's pocket or purse may be sufficient to allow the patient to ward off anticipatory anxiety which sometimes leads to panic. By the same token, knowledge that the therapist is available (perhaps with his or her telephone number in the pocket or purse) may serve the same preventive purpose. More intensive psychotherapy or behavioral treatment may be considered, but is rarely necessary and often not cost-effective. (See also Generalized Anxiety Disorder, below.)

300.02   Generalized Anxiety Disorder

The chronic presence of symptoms in the Generalized Anxiety Disorder make more careful treatment planning necessary, especially since the use of anxiolytic medication may have to be more extensive. The medication should be in sufficient dose to alleviate much of the painful anxiety but, as with Panic Disorder just discussed, formation of a therapeutic relationship will usually allow reassurance and the carrying of medications (or symbolic representations of the therapist) to supplant the chronic taking of drugs.

Brief psychotherapy for this condition may include acknowledgment (or even prediction) that the patient sometimes feels the anxiety will grow and grow until he or she is completely overwhelmed or feels in danger of "going crazy." It is often effective for the therapist to inform the patient that, although this condition is quite uncomfortable, it has predictable patterns (and is thus potentially understandable), and it is separate from the "psychotic" illnesses (and thus the patient will not "go crazy"). The possibility of frequent relapse should be frankly addressed as part of reassurance that the course of the disorder is fairly predictable and is likely to improve with time. As with Panic Disorder, intensive psychotherapy or psychoanalysis may be helpful for a few patients; however, it is usually not cost-effective unless there are clear underlying conflicts which the patient is motivated to address, and for which the patient can tolerate dynamic exploration.

Propranolol, which is effective for performance anxiety of various types, appears to be less effective for anxiety states or phobias. MAOIs and tricyclic antidepressants can block panic attacks in some patients; however, they should be reserved for those with refractory syndromes. Gorman et al. (1981) speak of the use of tricyclic antidepressants in the fairly large number of patients with Panic Disorder or Generalized Anxiety Disorder who have prolapsed mitral valves. The antidepressant does not appear to complicate the cardiac abnormality, which is generally felt to be benign. Propranolol has been suggested for such patients but evidence for success is lacking. Other medications which have been tried with limited success include clonidine (Hoehn-Saric et al., 1981) and alprazolam (*International Drug Therapy Newsletter*, 1981b). Rickels et al. (1980) mention the need for long-term follow-up of many of these patients, some of whom require continued medication.

Non-pharmacologic approaches for attenuating acute anxiety, and perhaps Panic Disorder, are often successful. Relaxation techniques, more specific behavioral treatment (e.g., biofeedback), or even regular transcendental meditation may be sufficient for many patients (see other parts of this section).

300.30 Obsessive Compulsive Disorder (or Obsessive Compulsive Neurosis)

The most effective treatment for uncomplicated obsessive compulsive disorder is exposure (in vivo, with or without fantasy). The in vivo treatments must include prevention of response (e.g., checking or washing). The clinician must be able to devote considerable session time to practice of the response prevention paradigm, discussion of the anxiety which appears when the response is prevented, and support when the anxiety dissipates. The treatment program should continue at home with the carefully orchestrated involvement of a family member or significant other. As with treatment of the phobias, continuing therapeutic support and counseling about the new "equilibrium" that will be experienced in a patient's life are important. Depression may appear as the symptoms wane, and can be treated with counseling and/or antidepressant medication (see below) as necessary (Marks, 1981b; Minchiello, 1981).

The only pharmacologic approach which has been reasonably useful is the use of clomipramine, a tricyclic antidepressant with clear anti-obsessional characteristics. This drug is not yet available in the U.S. but is expected to be marketed soon. Most studies indicate that it particularly addresses intrusive, unsettling obsessive thoughts, and that its effect on compulsive rituals may be significant as well. The hypothesis that it treats—either primarily or secondarily—underlying depression is inviting, but unproved (Insel, 1982; Marks et al., 1980). Other tricyclics may be tried, but results have been equivocal at best. Low doses of high potency neuroleptics (e.g., trifluoperazine 2 mg twice daily) have been used to disrupt obsessive compulsive symptoms, as have interruptions such as snapping a rubber band on the patient's wrist (when part of a behavioral program). Other medications are not particularly helpful. Traditional psychotherapy has in general not been effective by itself, although the here-and-now approaches appear more useful than analytic or psychodynamic therapies for most individuals.

It should be noted that in some patients obsessive compulsive symptoms defend against serious character psychology and the possibility of more severe disorganization. If careful evaluation reveals this underlying pathology, then straightforward behavioral treatment such as exposure should be undertaken with some caution, and the clinician should prepare to treat decompensation if it occurs. A few such patients show symptoms of bipolar disorder, and may benefit from inpatient observation and evaluation for lithium treatment.

308.30   Post-traumatic Stress Disorder, Acute

309.81   Post-traumatic Stress Disorder, Chronic or Delayed

Since these disorders may present with a variety of symptoms, often not primarily those of acute anxiety, a variety of treatment approaches should be considered depending upon patient need. Once the diagnosis is established, psychotherapeutic recognition of the dynamics and sympathy with the patient for having painful residuals of a traumatic event are useful. Discussion of the original trauma is helpful, and open examination of psychodynamic concepts such as survivor's guilt may provide a sort of cognitive structure with which the patient can view his or her experience in a more realistic light. Encouragement of normal and higher-order neurotic mechanisms for resolving the trauma will support those gains the patient has made. Conversely, subtly giving permission for the patient to continue to be disabled may delay improvement and strengthen unconscious secondary gain. Conveying to the patient the concept that he continues to be responsible for his life can be important in preventing unnecessary disability.

Temporary use of antianxiety or sleeping medication may be helpful. Low doses of diazepam at bedtime often suppress unwanted stage 4 non-REM sleep phenomena (some nightmares, night terrors, sleepwalking) (Reid et al., 1981, in press). Extended use of these medications is not recommended for most patients. Many of the principles of psychotherapy and medication of patients with Generalized Anxiety Disorder, discussed earlier, apply here.

In situations in which the disorder is chronic, and especially in which it is morbidly present, abreaction may be helpful. This may be done using hypnosis or chemically; however, most clinicians feel that sufficient abreaction can be attained without altering consciousness.

Some post-traumatic stress disorder patients, such as combat veterans or victims of mass disasters, benefit from lay support groups. Where possible, these should have the benefit of psychiatric consultation or participation.

300.00   Atypical Anxiety Disorder

The treatment of Atypical Anxiety Disorder should be predicated upon the symptoms presented and the underlying situational and psychodynamic issues elicited during the psychiatrist's evaluation. Many of the principles mentioned in this Anxiety Disorders section may apply. Pragmatic counseling in an atmosphere of support and reassurance is a good adjunct to any treatment program. For those patients whose anxiety is accompanied by considerable dependency or clinging to the therapist, specific rules for when and how the therapist will be available may alleviate some of the clinician's discomfort and provide an atmosphere of consistency for the patient.

Chapter 9

Somatoform Disorders

300.81 Somatization Disorder

The basic principle of definitive treatment of Somatization Disorder involves the removal of the emotional precursors of multiple medical complaints and/or the channeling of coping mechanisms for those precursors into behaviors or emotions which are more effective for the patient than are the symptoms of Somatization Disorder.

Most clinicians report only limited success for traditional psychodynamic intervention (Karasu, 1979; Kellner, 1975). Karasu recommends that the therapist relate to the patient as a physician to a medically ill individual, well informed about the patient's illness. Once this empathy and understanding have been established, a "life alliance" promotes friendly and educational interactions. After several weeks, the patient may eventually be able to explore feelings toward the therapist, feelings toward the somatic symptoms, and the possibility that these are related. Once the patient has meaningful insight into the relationships among affect, behavior, and somatization, symptoms of anxiety or physical distress should lessen (Karasu, 1979). Nevertheless, patients who express feelings in terms of bodily sensation may, by definition, be those who are reluctant to accept a psychiatric approach.

Group therapy may provide support and mild, tolerable confrontation for some patients. In this and individual therapy, the clinician should be alert for the appearance of non-somatic symptoms of underlying conflicts (e.g., depression), and be prepared to treat these accordingly.

Behavioral approaches, which are quite successful in changing specific behaviors and symptoms, have not been shown to have long-term usefulness in these disorders.

There is some evidence that continued medical contact short of major treatments such as surgery may be helpful. If the patient can be accepted by the physician, for example, secure in the anticipation of consistent brief visits to the doctor and attention to her (the patient is usually female) symptoms, the need for extraordinary interventions or escalation of symptoms may decrease.

300.11   Conversion Disorder (Hysterical Neurosis, Conversion Type)

There is considerable evidence that intensive or psychoanalytic psychotherapy is a useful treatment with patients with true hysterical neurosis. Unfortunately, patients with more severe underlying pathology (e.g., personality disorders) may appear clinically similar before treatment is begun. For those patients, dynamic psychotherapy may help with symptoms but is not the best approach in the long run.

The behavior therapies can, as in the case of many other disorders, remove symptoms. If this is the only goal of treatment, then behavior therapy or hypnosis should be considered. Both should be used in a broader context than mere symptom alleviation, with particular attention to techniques which increase the probability that improvement will be lasting, and will generalize to other maladaptive ways of handling the underlying conflicts involved in the symptom. In particular, hypnotic and other techniques which are sometimes misused to quickly "trick" the patient into losing his or her symptom should be avoided, except perhaps for diagnostic purposes. Such approaches tend to result in temporary improvement at best, and do a poor job of establishing the clinician as someone who has genuine respect for the patient and his or her difficulties.

Lazare (1981) notes that the psychiatrist may be of indirect assistance when conversion patients present in the general hospital setting by helping to differentiate conversion from organic symptoms or malingering, and by educating the hospital staff in methods of management and approaches to the patient (e.g., discouraging direct confrontation or accusations by staff).

Involvement of the spouse and/or other important family members in the patient's care, with an understanding of the social and psychodynamic issues that may be involved, can promote an atmosphere of better communication which may decrease the need for future conversion symptoms.

Patients with good premorbid adjustment, absence of major psychiatric syndromes, and the presence of a stressful event associated with acute onset of the conversion symptoms are associated with good prognosis. Most patients without severe underlying psychopathology continue to be significantly improved several years after treatment.

307.80   Psychogenic Pain Disorder

Getto and Ochitill (1982) note the benefit of viewing psychogenic pain (and indeed all chronic pain) multidimensionally. This biopsychosocial view places the psychiatrist within a multidisciplinary group of physicians and others, all of whom have the common goal of alleviating and preventing the patient's pain. One important aspect of this approach is that it may allow the patient to accept psychiatric intervention more readily, in a situation which the patient perceives as nonpsychiatric.

An important part of treatment is the clinician's belief that the patient actually feels pain and requires treatment. This—and the corollary belief that the patient is being honest with the physician—may have been lacking in many of the patient's earlier interactions with doctors.

One view of Psychogenic Pain Disorder compares it to other forms of chronic pain, and recommends treatment along similar lines. Specific pain clinics, usually found in larger medical institutions, use clear guidelines for evaluation, treatment goals, and attainment of goals. This structuring activity transforms a confusing and overwhelming experience into one which is broken down into manageable parts. The patient participates in the program to a great extent, and thereby gains some measure of mastery over feelings and sensations toward which he or she was formerly passive. The treatment programs are frequently behavioral in type, with reinforcement for decreasing "pain behavior" as well as for the more obvious goals of decreased use of medication and lessened perception of pain. Biofeedback is often used. Since the chronic pain takes place in, and is part of, the patient's family and social life, attention must be paid to education and counseling for the family and preparation for activities of ordinary daily living.

Such programs generally last for several weeks or months, and frequently have high success rates among patients who have not done well with previous (usually drug-oriented) regimens. The treatments are sometimes criticized for their emphasis on simply decreasing hospital visits and demands on the physician's time. Such goals should be seen as being attained because those behaviors are no longer necessary from the patient's point of view, and not as the result of punishment for visiting the clinic. Indeed, reassurance that the doctor and other means of alleviating pain are available is a large part of showing the patient that he or she does not need to use the medical facilities to prove that they are there.

The treatment of psychogenic pain and other forms of chronic pain with tricyclic antidepressants has been common for many years. While the best patient response often occurs at doses consistent with antidepressant activity, it has not been shown that the effectiveness of the medication is due to its antidepressant qualities. The tricyclics are recommended as an early choice, perhaps before resorting to inpatient programs; however, attention to the individual and family dynamics involved is imperative. Other medications, particularly the phenothiazines, and ECT have been recommended anecdotally but there are no good controlled studies to indicate that these should be early treatments of choice.

The psychiatrist who works with psychogenic pain, especially that which is an exaggeration of discomfort associated with existing medical illness, should be a person who works well within medical settings and is comfortable discussing and evaluating medical illness in his or her patients (Murphy & Davis, 1981). Many patients will be seen first in a consultation-liaison setting in the general hospital. Education of nursing staff and colleagues, along with practical suggestions for management of such concerns as patient anxiety, helplessness, or demandingness, will be indirectly helpful to the patient.

300.70   Hypochondriasis (or Hypochondriacal Neurosis)
In spite of many clinicians' wish not to reinforce hypochondriacal behavior, the psychiatrist must initially address the patient's physical condition and make some decision about its importance for the psychiatric treatment program. In some patients, a minority of those who fit DSM-III criteria for Hypochondriasis, discussing and explaining the negative results of a complete medical workup may bring relief. Taking time to educate the patient about the meaning of, for example, a referring internist's findings may provide knowledge and interest which will allow the hypochondriacal symptoms to subside.

Patients whose symptoms are more resilient may be successfully treated with a combination of psychotherapeutic and medical approaches. Kellner (1982a) noted considerable success with extended individual psychotherapy in which the patients were continually reminded of their selective perception that they were ill, shown that these perceptions were uncomfortable but physically innocuous, and given accurate information about medical symptoms and illnesses. Kellner and others feel that repeated physical examinations are a cost-effective way of reassuring patients.

Attention to the presence of other sources of anxiety and depression is important as well. Treatment of anxiety disorders (both chemically and psychotherapeutically) is discussed elsewhere in this volume, as is treatment of depressive illness.

In Hypochondriasis, and to some extent in Psychogenic Pain Disorder, concern over loss of the physician (and that which he or she symbolizes) can be a significant impediment to lasting improvement. Thus the physician who tells a patient, "I have good news. Your tests are all negative. You no longer need to see me," may precipitate further symptoms (in the case of pain) or complaints (in the case of Hypochondriasis) designed to recover the lost physician-object. A practical approach used by this author and recommended to nonpsychiatric colleagues is to convey to the patient that one is pleased that no dangerous illness is present (or that some recent illness has significantly improved), but that it is important that the patient practice good health habits and stay in contact with the doctor. This contact should be infrequent, so as to not engender unnecessary dependency or expense; however, it must be implied that the ongoing contact is *important*. The patient may, for example, be given a monthly 15-minute appointment and told "I know you may be feeling fine, but I want you to come in for a check-up without fail."

Traditional insight-oriented psychotherapy is indicated for those patients whose hypochondriasis is particularly pervasive and is symptomatic of conflicts which are likely to be responsive to this mode of treatment. Once the patient has entered psychodynamic psychotherapy, it may be useful to discourage talk about the hypochondriacal symptoms during certain phases of treatment, with the idea that this topic is one of resistance and prevents the surfacing of other important material. Some patients, after several months, describe their symptoms as having subtly disappeared, while they were unaware that they were decreasing in intensity.

300.70   Atypical Somatoform Disorder

Treatment of Atypical Somatoform Disorders should be based upon the presenting symptoms and the clinician's understanding of their underlying causes.

Chapter 10

Dissociative Disorders (Hysterical Neuroses, Dissociative Type)

300.12 Psychogenic Amnesia

Perhaps the most common dissociative disorder which comes to medical attention is Psychogenic Amnesia. It may present in a medical setting (e.g., emergency room), certain vocational settings (e.g., military), or following severe psychic trauma (which may be accompanied by physical injury). Treatment should begin as early as possible, since the amnesia may stabilize in time and be further incorporated into the patient's emotional structure.

Both active and passive treatment methods have been advocated. Since amnesia produces anxiety in family and friends (often more than in the patient), there is usually pressure to alleviate it quickly. Amytal or thiopental interviews and hypnotic techniques have an excellent probability of access to the suppressed memories of psychogenic retrograde amnesia. The suggestion may be made that the patient will recall the events upon arousal; however, many clinicians prefer to allow the patient to make this decision, saying something like: "When you become alert you will be able to remember as much of our interview as you like; the rest will come to you with time, when you are ready to recall it." This allows the mind to use the amnesia for its intended, defensive purpose while eliminating as much of the symptom as is practical. Amphetamines have been used in barbiturate interviews to stimulate patients' productions. There is no clear evidence that this is due to any particular anamnestic property of the stimulants. It seems more likely that the addition of small amounts of I.V. amphetamine titrate the level of consciousness and allow more verbal interchange.

Another approach, which may be used alone or in combination with the rapid symptom removal mentioned above, is that of providing a supportive environment in which the psyche may allow its barriers to be lowered. In some such settings, a long, supportive interview in which the patient is asked to discuss at length the memories, associations, and feelings which come to mind may be all that is necessary. In others, the memory returns over a period of days or weeks of support and gentle reminders. In this light, dependency itself is not to be encouraged; brief psychotherapy may be aimed at helping the patient to find defenses other than amnesia with which he or she can cope with the emotionally stressful event that precipitated the symptoms.

300.13 Psychogenic Fugue
Psychogenic Fugue may be considered similar in purpose to amnesia but as involving a necessity for more dissociation from an affect-laden event and/or from the self. Many of the treatment techniques described above for Psychogenic Amnesia are useful for Fugue. The clinician should expect treatment to be more lengthy, consistent with the more massive defensive mechanism (and/or consistent with the premorbid character structure which was predisposed to it). Since Psychogenic Fugue may last longer than amnesia, therapeutic strategies which include more intense psychodynamic therapy are often suggested. At the least, a continuing supportive relationship with a psychotherapist is recommended for preventing future episodes of dissociation.

Caution is in order with respect to the use of intensive hypnotic techniques in patients with Psychogenic Amnesia or Psychogenic Fugue. Research by a number of clinicians, notably Orne (1979), indicate that what may appear to be restitution of old memory is often actually construction of new "memory." In most patients this is not problematic; however, when the recovering of a specific memory from the past is important (for legal reasons, for example), hypnosis should be used with the greatest of care in order to assure that the "memory" is not actually an iatrogenic confabulation which has been permanently embedded in the patient's perception of the past.

300.14 Multiple Personality
The treatment of Multiple Personality is far more complex and lengthy than that of the above, relatively encapsulated syndromes. This condition should not be considered synonymous with schizophreniform or schizophrenic disorders, and should not be treated with antipsychotic medication unless indi-

cated by the symptoms presented. The traditional treatment approach, popularized by Thigpen and Cleckley (1957), is intensely psychodynamic or psychoanalytic, often aided by hypnosis (Bowers, 1971). The hypnotic portion of treatment may be used to uncover material for therapeutic exploration outside the trance or, if the clinician is trained in the psychoanalytic use of trance, may be an aid to restructuring the patient's character in such a way as to integrate the various separated parts ("multiple personalities"), each of which is incomplete without the others.

The psychotherapeutic treatment of Multiple Personality requires sufficient subspecialization that the clinician should either be experienced in this area or seek supervision. The patient (who presents as several people, only some of whom may see "themselves" as "patients") will tend to be quite demanding and frustrating.

As with the amnestic and fugue states, the legal implications of Multiple Personality may be significant to the treatment process. Unconscious secondary gain at the level of dependency needs may interfere with analytic attempts to reach the deeper defensive purposes of the disintegration of the self.

300.60   Depersonalization Disorder (Depersonalization Neurosis)

Nemiah (1980) provides an elegant description of the clinical features of Depersonalization Disorder which are relevant to its treatment and prognosis. He notes that the disorder tends to be chronic, but that many patients experience long periods without symptoms of depersonalization. The association of acute anxiety with onset (or reemergence) of symptoms suggests that many of the treatment approaches for acute and chronic anxiety (q.v.) may be helpful in the management of symptomatic periods of Depersonalization Disorder.

Although feelings of unreality may sound "psychotic," the condition appears clinically (and biochemically) unrelated to the thought disorders, an observation which is consistent with the lack of success of chronic neuroleptic medication. Access to the source of the depersonalization symptom, for diagnostic purposes or to provide the clinician with material for psychotherapy, may be gotten through barbiturate interviews or (in some cases) hypnosis; however, these do not appear to have lasting therapeutic value.

The patient is usually quite aware of the dissociative episodes. In those situations in which some belle indifference is present, many clinicians would speak of Briquet's Syndrome and apply treatment measures related to those for hysteria. In other patients, however, the depersonalization is quite frightening.

The assumption that Depersonalization Disorder represents a severe neurosis (perhaps a "character neurosis") makes analytically oriented psychotherapy a consideration. The depth of psychopathology in persons with severe depersonalization has been seen by some as a contraindication to psychoanalysis; however, recent progress in the fields of analysis of character disorders and disorders of the self should cause the clinician to consider consultation with, or referral to, a qualified analyst.

300.15 Atypical Dissociative Disorder

Treatment of patients with dissociative symptoms which do not fit any of the above DSM-III categories should focus upon the symptoms and syndromes as they present, and upon the apparent underlying psychopathology. The presence of dissociation ordinarily suggests a massive defensive effort which, in turn, suggests a relatively acute trauma (which has rekindled earlier conflicts by virtue either of the strength of the conflict or the strength of the trauma). For those patients with relatively good premorbid functioning and/or well encapsulated symptoms, a symptomatic approach is likely to be helpful. One example might be the treatment of some forms of sleepwalking (somnambulism). Many such patients, after sleepwalking as children, will be free of the symptom until some external stress appears in an otherwise uneventful life (e.g., an important loss). Treatment approaches described by Reid et al. (in press) indicate that symptom removal can occur without psychodynamic complications.

Chapter 11

Psychosexual Disorders

GENDER IDENTITY DISORDERS

302.5x Transsexualism

In recent years the physician's ability to accommodate—endocrinologically and/or surgically—the transsexual's desire to become a member of the opposite sex has occupied a central position in clinical and popular concepts of the treatment of this disorder. Such a simplistic view is unjustified, however, in spite of the yearnings and demands which may come from patients who identify themselves to the psychiatrist as transsexual. After the diagnosis has been made, and differentiation from Transvestism (302.30) and Ego-dystonic Homosexuality (302.00) has been established, extensive evaluation and counseling are necessary before irreversible and potentially dangerous procedures should be undertaken.

Virtually every study on this topic recommends a long period (generally over one year) of psychotherapy prior to any decision for surgical reassignment of sex. This treatment is not to "talk the patient out of it"; rather it is to help the patient develop insight, understand him/herself and the potential outcomes of his/her therapeutic plans, and realistically appraise his/her future. At this time the therapist should support the patient, and search for areas of conflict for which some avenue of relief of anxiety other than surgery may be acceptable to the patient.

During this period, male or female hormones can be administered, preferably under the supervision of an endocrinologist. Green (1982) makes the important observation that although most or all of the effects of female hormones on males are reversible, some of the effects of androgens on females are not.

Keller et al. (1982) noted that group therapy can be an ideal setting for the treatment, observation, and evaluation of gender-dysphoric patients before, during, and after surgery. Those authors reported that 43% of patients in analytically oriented group psychotherapy elected nonsurgical solutions. Other reports regarding the psychotherapeutic or psychoanalytic treatment of the gender identity disorders are less optimistic about their ability to effectively resolve basic conflicts and decrease patients' discomfort in any lasting way. This is not meant to apply to psychotherapy designed to assist patients in accepting or adapting to situations related to their transsexualism (see below.)

"Success rates" for sex reassignment surgery must be viewed with caution (Lothstein, 1982). The characteristics of follow-up studies, even those which are long-term, make comparison difficult. For males, dissatisfaction with some aspect of sex reassignment (physical, social, religious, or other) is common, although most persons who have had the surgery are glad that they did. Virtually all authors consider the surgery as a last resort for a select group of patients.

Far fewer female than male transsexuals have had sex change operations, in spite of similar numbers of individuals who describe themselves as transsexuals among both sexes. The surgical procedures for females at the present time are less satisfactory than those for males, and more problems after surgery appear to occur in genetically female patients. In spite of these problems, Sorensen (1981) reports that, like males, few females regretted having the operation(s).

The postsurgical adaptation of the patient is of extreme importance. Issues of self-image must be addressed. In addition, attempts to normalize the social and interpersonal lives of these patients, and perhaps to help them separate from the quasi-supportive world of those who are less successfully struggling with their sexual disorders, involve extensive support, understanding, education, and insight. Problems with families in whom the transsexual is a parent are particularly difficult. Children have serious problems coping with role changes of this magnitude, and deserve special attention themselves.

Sorensen (1981) and others have noted that the prognosis for transsexuals who have surgery is considerably better for those patients who have a stable life-style before sex change and fewer signs of other forms of severe psychopathology. Those who have the greatest expectations for surgery and the most demanding fantasies regarding it tend to be far less satisfied.

Nonsurgical approaches other than intensive psychotherapy (e.g., behavioral programs) have generally had poor results vis-à-vis a treatment goal of changing the transsexual orientation. Various other forms of psychotherapy may be of considerable use in alleviating some of the pain attendant to the condition.

302.60   Gender Identity Disorder of Childhood
Issues related to this disorder, which may be closely related to the development of adult gender identity disorders or other sexual problems, are discussed in the section on Disorders Usually First Evident in Infancy, Childhood, or Adolescence.

302.85   Atypical Gender Identity Disorder
The treatment of these residual syndromes should be based upon presenting symptoms and underlying psychiatric disorders or issues. Much caution should be exercised before embarking on broad and/or irreversible treatment programs, since the placing of patients in this category may be based more upon a clinician's intuition or anecdotal experience than upon the meeting of established criteria for, for example, sex reassignment surgery.

PARAPHILIAS
There are a number of general treatment considerations which can be discussed as common to many of the paraphilias. The psychiatrist or other mental health professional called upon to treat these patients must have a therapeutic orientation rather than a punitive one, and must be comfortable with his or her own feelings regarding these often criminal patients (particularly those of a more exploitive or aggressive nature). Serious manifestations of countertransference will almost certainly arise and must be understood and managed.

From a practical, if not always a psychodynamic viewpoint, distinction should be drawn between those paraphilias which do not intrude upon the wishes of others (e.g., Fetishism, Transvestism), those which intrude but are nonviolent (e.g., Exhibitionism, Voyeurism), and those which are not only intrusive but seriously aggressive or otherwise potentially injurious to others (e.g., Sexual Sadism, Pedophilia). The treatment of patients with sexually oriented disorders which are more properly described as aggressive (e.g., rapists) is addressed to some extent in this section, but the sections on Personality Disorders and Adult Antisocial Behavior should also be consulted (see pp. 187, 201).

Treatment may be requested by those who are uncomfortable with their paraphilic orientation, by those whose family or social situations do not tolerate the paraphilia (and for whom the paraphilia is less important to maintain than the family or social environment), or by the patient for whom the community demands change because of some criminal activity. In the latter case, important issues of motivation, coercion, and treatment against one's will come into play. It is this author's feeling that patients anticipating trial on criminal charges are usually not good candidates for long-term treatment decisions; however, once the case has been settled in some way, those patients who remain in treatment often have a good prognosis.

The presence of paraphilic behavior is often associated—by patient or clinician—with some transient stress. If the disorder is clearly chronic, the therapist should take care not to allow the patient to rationalize or devalue the importance of the symptom with statements such as, "The job pressures were too great," or "I understand now that the whole thing happened because my wife was pregnant." On the other hand, for those patients for whom insight-oriented psychotherapy is appropriate, considerable effort should be made to explore the paraphilic behavior as symptomatic of conflict (and thus as explorable by clinician and patient) rather than as a heinous and irreversible part of the patient's personality. Even though many of these conditions are refractory to many forms of treatment, punitive attitudes for punishment's sake have no place in the treatment program.

No matter what form of treatment is chosen, many authors recommend some level of participation of the patient's family. Kentsmith and Eaton (1979) particularly recommend counseling of spouses, conjoint therapy, and/or participation of the spouse as a co-therapist in various treatment programs. This not only helps the patient, but allays anxieties and increases the spouse's acceptance of the patient and treatment program.

Removal of paraphilic symptoms often leads to the surfacing of other problems in the patient's life. These may range from interpersonal difficulties (e.g., marital problems), to anxiety related to conflicts which were being defended against by the paraphilic behavior, to previously undiagnosed depression. Treatment for these conditions is discussed elsewhere.

302.81   Fetishism

The treatment of Fetishism rarely involves concerns about criminality or danger to others. Presenting complaints generally revolve around guilt or difficulty with one's sexual partner. If the complaint is mild, education about the condition and its benign course may alleviate the patient's anxiety about, for example, whether his symptom indicates deep-seated mental illness. It is necessary that the therapist be comfortable with this sort of giving of "permission" for the patient to practice his sexual preference. In those situations in which the guilt is more significant, the patient recognizes the fetishistic symptom as only one of a constellation of neurotic symptoms, and/or the fetishism interferes with desired or necessary activities in other spheres, more intensive treatment is needed.

Although behavioral techniques may remove the symptoms, this author prefers psychodynamically oriented treatment aimed either at resolution of underlying conflicts or at development of more efficient ego defenses. Once this approach to treatment is undertaken, it is important that the therapist not ally himself or herself with the symptom-producing portion of the patient's ego. Thus, although the symptom should be seen as neither good nor bad, it must be confronted as something which the patient him/herself has labeled undesirable. This is particularly true if the fetishism has led to some sort of mild criminal activity such as stealing women's underclothing.

Treatment often involves the patient's sexual partner, and indeed this is imperative if the presentation is one of marital difficulty or rejection of the sexual behavior by a spouse. Education is important and should take place in a conjoint setting if possible. Spouses (or patients) who complain loudly that the fetishistic behavior is intractable or ruining the relationship can often be found to be scapegoating the paraphilia. In such cases, complete treatment necessitates a serious attempt by all involved to uncover other, often nonsexual issues which may be contributing to the couple's difficulties.

302.30   Transvestism

Although Transvestism may superficially resemble Transsexualism and/or Homosexuality in its presentation, it is more properly considered for treatment among disorders such as Fetishism. In this light, many of the principles just outlined for treatment of fetishists may be applied to transvestites. Since the symptoms are more visible (to both the patient and to others), probably less common, and require more effort to carry out, the issues of anxiety, guilt, social difficulty, and family (especially spousal) dissatisfaction are usually more prominent. The ability of the treating clinician to be comfortable "giving permission" for the activity may be less than in Fetishism. The likelihood of the patient's accepting an extensive treatment plan (at least for those persons who consult a psychiatrist at all) is probably higher than for fetishists. The social association of Transvestism with Homosexuality and Transsexualism frequently adds an important dimension to problems with relationships, that of the patient's need to assert to himself his masculinity, his heterosexuality, or perhaps to play out some perceived prophecy of homosexuality.

The clinician should not confuse treatment of Transvestism with that of Transsexualism. The use of hormones, and especially of surgery, has no place in the management of this disorder.

302.10 Zoophilia

As with the previous two disorders, education, handling of anxiety, and alleviation of guilt are important for the treatment of the dysphoric aspects of Zoophilia. In some cases, the patient may (as in the previous conditions) leave the clinician's care and continue with his symptom, minus the anxieties which brought him to treatment. In others, alleviation of some of the anxieties and concomitant increase in self-image may allow the patient to tolerate psychotherapeutic exploration of the symptom, with the goal of its eventual demise. This is particularly important when symptoms such as Zoophilia, Fetishism, Exhibitionism, and the like are part of depressive syndromes in which the guilt that one feels after the sexual act, the feeling of being a sexual deviate, or the embarrassment of being caught may be seen as both symptomatic and self-destructive.

In the case of Zoophilia it is particularly important that the therapist have some knowledge of the differential probability of sexual behavior with animals among various patient groups. For example, adolescent sexual experience with farm animals in rural settings is far more common than, say, intercourse with animals among persons raised in urban settings. By the same token, this paraphilia is more likely than many of the others to be seen in both men and women.

The therapist should also be able to educate, and perhaps treat, the patient with respect to disease acquired in connection with Zoophilia. While ordinary venereal diseases are not transmissible across most species, a number of other medical complications may arise.

Finally, this paraphilia, like some of the others to be discussed, involves an aspect of exploitation or even cruelty in some of its manifestations. Issues of sadism and masochism should be explored when therapeutically possible.

302.20 Pedophilia

A famous philosopher, upon his second arrest and lengthy sentence for Pedophilia, was once asked why he returned so quickly to the behavior when he knew his punishment would be so severe. He replied, in effect, "Because it is worth it." This statement seems to reflect the intractability of Pedophilia, an intractability which is sometimes common to the other paraphilias but which, for a variety of reasons, seems more prominent in those who molest children.

Treatment of the disorder is often complicated, or even constrained, by the presence of legal conditions such as probation, incarceration, or loss of custody of one's children. In some cases these are used to advantage, for example as motivating factors and barriers to denial; in others, society's legitimate needs to protect its children interfere with such basic components of treatment as voluntariness and confidentiality. Ethical and legal decisions regarding breach of confidentiality to protect potential victims must sometimes be made.

The principles of psychotherapeutic treatment, except for not giving the patient permission to continue the symptoms, are similar to those for the other paraphilias, but the insight-oriented psychotherapies are not well accepted for this disorder. Once the patient has become visible, society demands more rapid, observable modes of treatment, which can be given under at least a semblance of social control. There is a psychodynamic assumption of immature or improperly fixated sexual choice, whether because of basic defects in development per se or because of regression based upon underlying depression, organic impairment, or other cardinal psychopathology.

The social magnitude of the activity being greater than that of any of the previously discussed paraphilias, the opportunity for denial, guilt, self-castigation, marital problems, and the like is greater. It should be especially noted that the possibility of suicide after discovery of pedophilic activity is significant, particularly in a professional person or one who is highly visible in the community. This is true as well, but to a lesser extent, for public discovery of any of the other paraphilias.

Behavioral conditioning, primarily aversive, is the most widely used treatment approach. Various success rates are reported; these usually are optimistic for the first few months (especially while the patient is either in treatment or under legal scrutiny such as bond or probation). Aversive techniques have included electric shock and induction of vomiting. Social movements away from the more painful aversive therapies have led to the development of milder shock conditioning and to the use of the technique of snapping a rubber band against one's skin (which can be done either by a therapist or by the patient himself). Recent emphasis has moved to some extent from passive aversion therapy to self-management programs (including self-administration of aversion) and sexual skills training (Marks, 1981a). Marks cites the use of fading as another method of decreasing deviant sexual stimuli. In this approach, subjects are gradually shifted toward more conventional sexual content during periods of sexual arousal, either in fantasy, by using visual (e.g., photographic) techniques, or by conditioning orgasm.

Biological reduction of sexual drive is often recommended for Pedophilia. Although there is a lack of adequately controlled studies which address the extent to which physical castration actually reduces male sexual approach behavior, some authors recommend orchydectomy in cases of unmanageable and dangerous (e.g., pedophilic or sadistic) paraphilias (Freund, 1980). Stereotaxic procedures are theoretically promising, but not appropriate for clinical use at this time.

A method of sex drive reduction which is more palatable to western culture is antiandrogenic medication. The most common agents currently in use are cyproterone acetate and medroxyprogesterone acetate (MPA). Both of these are effective in controlling cases of deviant hypersexuality and paraphilia by reducing libido and overt sexual behavior. The advantages of these pharmacologic means of reducing circulating plasma testosterone include: A medical rather than punitive posture is taken; the effects appear to be reversible in most cases; some secondary sex characteristics and even some appropriate sexual impulses and behavior may be preserved in many patients; and the ability to obtain consent for the treatment (from patient, institution, and/ or appropriate governmental agency) is far greater than might be the case for orchydectomy or neurosurgery (Berlin & Meinecke, 1981; Gagné, 1981; Herrmann & Beach, 1980). MPA can be given in depot form; noncompliance is the major reason for return of symptoms. Cyproterone acetate is preferred by many Canadian and European clinical researchers (Bradford, 1982).

Important clinical and social decisions remain about whether to allow many of these highly recidivistic patients to live in the community while they are being treated. Family, social, and vocational problems, continuing superficial and deep emotional difficulties, and the temptation to deny one's disorder (and thus quit the medication) after the symptoms have abated make continuing psychotherapy imperative for these patients.

302.40 Exhibitionism

Outpatient treatment of Exhibitionism has probably received more attention in the literature than that of any other paraphilia. The resistance of the symptom to change, either with treatment or with time, approaches that of Pedophilia, although it is far less intrusive or exploitive for its victims. Treatment methods which have been employed, sometimes with considerable success, include behavioral approaches such as those already discussed (Blair & Lanyon, 1981). Individual psychotherapy can be useful for those patients who fill the usual criteria for psychodynamic work, provided motivation continues and denial is not allowed to exert too great a resistive influence. Behavioral treatment for short-term improvement (which may lead to strengthening of the self-image or to dysphoria as conflicts are expressed by other means) may offer a foundation on which ongoing therapy can be built.

Group psychotherapy has been a common approach, with a number of anecdotal reports of success. Participation or co-treatment of spouses of exhibitionists is advocated by many (Bastani & Kentsmith, 1980). Specialized hypnotherapeutic strategies have often been reported for this and other paraphilias (Mutter, 1981), but conclusive evidence of response is lacking. Simple hypnotic suggestion alone is useless. Treatment approaches which focus upon the situational components of exhibitionism and other impulsive paraphilic behaviors, which often appear strikingly obsessive and anxiety-related, may be helpful (Snaith & Collins, 1981); however, controlled studies are lacking.

The use of antiandrogenic drugs (cyproterone acetate or medroxyprogesterone acetate) has been advocated in intractable exhibitionism and more severe forms of other nonviolent paraphilias. Such recommendations cite the drug's apparent reversibility, acceptance by patients, frequent legal (and often vocational and family) complications of exhibitionistic behavior, and the presence of dysphoria which is often greater than that seen in, for example, fetishists. This author would reserve consideration of antiandrogenic treatments for a last resort, being especially cautious to rule out the presence of underlying major affective disorder which is treatable by other means.

302.82   Voyeurism
The symptoms of the true voyeur are often as resistant as those of the exhibitionist, although his dangerousness to society and intrusiveness upon those around him may be less. Treatment approaches are similar to those for paraphilias such as exhibitionism. Family, social, and legally-related considerations are likewise important. This author would tend not to recommend antiandrogenic treatment for patients whose primary disorder is voyeurism in the absence of accompanying chronic symptoms of violence, exploiting of children, or intractable hypersexuality.

302.83   Sexual Masochism
The treatment of Sexual Masochism per se, which is now known to be much less a disorder of women than was once thought, is (like that of many of the other paraphilias) actually the treatment of those masochistic persons who come to clinical attention. There is little in the literature about treatment, although much discussion and many case reports exist in the psychodynamic and psychoanalytic literature on the topic of masochism in general. The clinical cases described may not approximate the DSM-III diagnosis.

Superficial symptomatic treatment with such methods as assertiveness training, bolstering of self-image and self-worth, and the like may be helpful for some patients, for example those who have in the past accepted a victim role but are no longer satisfied with it. If the clinician's evaluation reveals roots of the masochism in depression, ennui, or existential apathy, then specific treatment for these (psychotherapeutic and/or pharmacologic) may be helpful.

More intensive psychotherapy, aimed at discovering and resolving causative conflicts and/or developing more efficient, less destructive defense mechanisms, is indicated for those patients who can utilize and tolerate this approach. The therapist will frequently be reminded that this sexual behavior, like the other paraphilias, will retain its gratifying value for long periods and will be available to the patient during times of regression.

302.84   Sexual Sadism

Once this disorder has been differentiated from primarily violent, quasi-sexual behaviors, decisions regarding treatment may be divided into two approaches, both of which are little addressed in the literature. For those patients who inflict physical or emotional suffering on nonconsenting others, especially when the disorder is not marked by dysphoria at some time, the social and legal issues discussed earlier in the sections on Pedophilia and Exhibitionism become important. Society may dictate control, prescribe certain treatments, or constrain other treatment approaches, as already discussed. The use of antiandrogenic medication may be necessary and should be considered when the protection of others is an issue; however, in the absence of dysphoria (at least discomfort induced by threat of arrest, unemployment, or divorce), adequate consent may be impossible to obtain.

For those patients who practice sexual sadism with a consenting partner, the presence of dysphoria during some phase (e.g., between sexual activities, just after orgasm) or threat of family loss may bring the patient to treatment. Behavioral approaches similar to those already discussed are worthy of consideration (e.g., the fading technique described by Marks [1981b]).

In some instances, a partner may receive severe or permanent injury. Such cases usually indicate severe psychopathology in both partners, and necessitate protection of the victim even if "consent" is present. It goes without saying that this issue is all the more important when it involves persons legally unable to consent (e.g., minors, elderly or incompetent individuals, or patients in institutions for the retarded or mentally ill). In such situations, control of the sadist must be part of treatment.

302.90   Atypical Paraphilia

The treatment of individuals who fall into this residual category should be predicated upon their presenting symptoms and underlying psychopathology. The extent to which treatment should be vigorously pursued by the clinician, and to which the more invasive therapies (e.g., antiandrogenic drugs) should be used, depends in large measure upon how intrusive or injurious the paraphilia is for persons other than the patient, upon the depth of dysphoria attached to the symptoms, and upon the magnitude of the social and legal implications of the repeated paraphilic behavior.

PSYCHOSEXUAL DYSFUNCTIONS

The treatment of the Psychosexual Dysfunctions has been extensively discussed by a number of authors, from a variety of clinical points of view. The well-known and often highly successful Masters and Johnson techniques will be briefly touched upon, but are described in more detail elsewhere (Masters & Johnson, 1970). It should be noted that superficial knowledge of these and other treatment modalities is insufficient for their successful use. Specialized training, clinical experience, and attention to one's own emotional reactions are all recommended.

Graber (1981) suggests that most physicians and psychotherapists with legitimate clinical interests can assume a role in the treatment of specific sexual dysfunctions. Marmor (1982), however, notes that psychiatrists tend to see patients who have already been to other therapists, and thus may be those with deeper problems or those who are more difficult to treat. Other authors have reviewed the behavioral psychotherapy of sexual disorders (e.g., Marks, 1981b), other short-term treatments (Cooper, 1981), and the necessity for psychodynamic exploration in many patients who present with complaints of sexual dysfunction (Marmor, 1982).

Several of the DSM-III Psychosexual Dysfunctions fall under the rubric of disorders of desire, excitement, or orgasm. Patients with disorders of sexual desire tend to have deeper psychopathological reasons for the conditions, and may benefit most from psychodynamic or psychoanalytic treatment (although situational factors, particularly in those patients in whom the symptoms are of recent onset, are also important). Disorders of orgasm, on the other hand, are more likely to be successfully treated behaviorally (or with other short-term approaches) in spite of the presence of psychodynamic factors. Limited treatment objectives, often aimed at single dysfunctional symptoms, may eliminate the complaint. Simple removal of the sexual dysfunction may be a catalyst for growth in other areas of one's self and the relationships involved; however, more comprehensive approaches, often involving the sexual partner as well, are usually indicated.

In spite of great temptation to treat individuals and couples on an outpatient basis within the traditional once-a-week context, the original Masters and Johnson recommendation for two or more weeks of daily, intensive work has stood the test of time. This approach tests the motivation of the couple, may weed out many patients for whom the treatment may be less successful, establishes the dedication of both partners to the importance of their sexual relationship and their marriage, fosters an intensive immersion in the treatment method which would otherwise be diluted by the many days between treatment sessions, and allows improvement over a period of days or weeks rather than months or years.

H. S. Kaplan (1979) discusses the indications for various kinds of treatment including, but not limited to, specialized sex therapy. She and other authors sometimes disagree about the place of psychotropic medications in the treatment of psychosexual dysfunction per se; however, the use of drugs in the treatment of complicating underlying disorders such as depression or disorganized thinking is generally accepted. The side effects of such medications, some of which involve changes in energy level, libido, and genital physiology (e.g., secretions, ejaculation), must be considered.

302.71   Inhibited Sexual Desire

Disorders of this phase of sexual activity require greater consideration of (particularly psychodynamic) psychotherapy than do the other dysfunctions. Nevertheless, ascertaining that the patient has accurate and relevant *information* about sexuality in general, his or her personal sexual activity, and (often overlooked) reproductive issues is an important first step. Nonthreatening but matter-of-fact history-taking, with attention to those feelings and activities which are avoided or suppressed in the interview, should follow. These represent the beginning of the therapeutic relationship and desensitization of the patient, no matter what the eventual treatment plan.

The prescribing of highly structured tasks, in an authoritative manner, should then take place, using techniques similar to those recommended by Kaplan (1979) and/or Masters and Johnson (1970). These tasks explore the giving and receiving of pleasure, development of the ability to fantasize, comfort with the sharing of sexual experiences with one's partner, and broader issues of the relationship between the partners.

Treatment should be provided in an atmosphere which can offer consistent and multifaceted attention not only to the symptom, but also to accompanying and peripheral feelings and behaviors.

302.72   Inhibited Sexual Excitement

Although more physically visible and anxiety-producing in males, the increasing ability of women to recognize Inhibited Sexual Excitement as something which interferes with pleasure (and the availability of treatment techniques) brings individuals of both sexes to seek treatment.

In males, the concept of "performance anxiety" has been well established and has led to treatment settings in which sexual stimulation is present but demands (or perceived demands) for performance are minimized. Various levels of "pleasuring" are prescribed by the (preferably conjoint) therapist(s), to take place in uninterrupted privacy. At first, there is a proscription against genital stimulation; later it is allowed, but orgasm is avoided. An escalating hierarchy of brief, followed by extended, sexual contacts (including intercourse) then takes place, in a manner identical to the behavioral concept of desensitization, with each step designed to create as little opportunity for "failure" as possible (e.g., making initial physical contact brief). A similar approach is often effective for women who have psychogenic difficulty attaining or maintaining labial and vaginal preparation for intercourse (e.g., lubrication).

In both men and women, these symptomatic treatments should not be carried out without the availability of additional, adjunctive measures to address educational, psychotherapeutic, and sometimes religious needs.

302.73   Inhibited Female Orgasm

Both psychodynamic and behavioral approaches to the treatment of Inhibited Female Orgasm stress the lowering of barriers to the releasing aspect of sexual climax. Traditional psychotherapeutic methods of addressing excessive control (or fear of being out of control) have been generally unsatisfactory. Education and specific training, regarding clitoral stimulation or pubococcygeal control (Graber, 1982), for example, are often very useful. A single therapist may be recommended, particularly a woman.

Group therapy has been advocated, in which discussions of masturbatory techniques and further "permission" are fostered. Kaplan (1974) discusses the importance of "distracting" the patient and the use of erotic paraphernalia. The employing of masturbation may extend beyond manual stimulation to vibrators, running water, or other objects. Their judicious use carries few or no dangers, despite occasional comments in the literature about "dependence" upon mechanical aids.

It is important to note that the complaint of anorgasmia may be a limited one, in which orgasm with masturbation is present but orgasm with one's partner (or one particular partner) is absent. In such instances, the patient may or may not fill criteria for a DSM-III diagnosis of Inhibited Female Orgasm. Initial evaluation should ascertain whether the anorgasmia is based upon differences in a partner's sexual technique, upon characteristics of the relationship with a partner, or upon emotional characteristics concerning relationships in general (e.g., allowing oneself to trust or share pleasure with the other person during a time of intimacy and vulnerability). These are all issues whose treatment should be approached at the appropriate level of education, counseling, or insight-oriented psychotherapy.

302.74 Inhibited Male Orgasm

Many characteristics of treatment of Inhibited Male Orgasm are similar to those for Inhibited Female Orgasm, just discussed. The likelihood of educational or simple counseling approaches being effective seems somewhat lower for men since orgasm is an extremely common experience for most males in most cultures, and since the reproductive function of ejaculation is closely associated with male orgasm. Psychogenic inhibition of male orgasm, then, is likely to reflect a condition for which exploration of psychodynamic issues is indicated. Nevertheless, education, "permission," and behavioral approaches should be tried, particularly if the sexual history indicates that these may be of use. As noted earlier, intensive psychotherapy is not the only route to change and growth within the psyche; symptomatic change, particularly within an area of such emotional importance as sexual dysfunction, may provide the beginning of growth in many other spheres of the patient's life and self.

Relative inhibition of male orgasm, such as that found in individuals who require extraordinarily long periods of stimulation or intercourse before ejaculation occurs, may be of concern to the patient and to the partner, who may be not only inconvenienced, but also made uncomfortable. Desensitization exercises which employ manual stimulation prior to intromission are generally useful, often combined with the providing of additional stimulation during intercourse. The latter may come from fantasy, erotic paraphernalia or vibrators, or, perhaps most commonly, from the partner in the form of stroking, anal stimulation, particular kinds of thrusting, or sexual conversation. "Distraction" techniques may also be used.

302.75 Premature Ejaculation

Premature Ejaculation is the sexual dysfunction most associated with complete, successful treatment by behavioral means. The well-known "squeeze" technique, in which the female partner stimulates the penis almost to orgasm and then prevents orgasm and ejaculation with firm pressure below the glans is an effective, hierarchical desensitization method. It is now widely accepted that the squeezing itself is not always necessary; the male partner can merely tell the woman when he is near orgasm, she stops stimulating him, the sexual feelings are allowed to dissipate, and the process is repeated. As with the squeeze technique, after several repetitions the couple move a step closer to intercourse, perhaps by adding the use of a lubricant. Later the start-and-stop activity is done with the penis inside the vagina, with the woman controlling movements and stopping when ejaculation is near. As the hierarchy progresses, male thrusting is allowed only until a sensation of loss of control is felt; later, other positions are used. The similarity between this and other desensitization techniques in which "failure" is not allowed to occur is obvious, and is extremely important for the success of treatment.

302.76   Functional Dyspareunia

Functional Dyspareunia may be approached in a manner similar to that of Somatization Disorder (300.81; page 147), in that it is a physiologic manifestation of emotional conflict. As with the Somatoform Disorders, the pain is—for the patient—an effective means of dealing with an unacceptable fear or impulse. With this in mind, approaches to treatment should consider psychodynamic issues, and may include insight-oriented psychotherapy.

Behavioral approaches which employ gentle, non-pressured, perhaps graduated attempts at stimulation, orgasm, and intercourse are recommended; however, informal attempts at this are likely already to have been tried by the patient-couple. It is thus important that such an approach take place in a professional context, accompanied by individual or conjoint psychotherapy.

306.51   Functional Vaginismus

As is the case in Functional Dyspareunia, Functional Vaginismus is likely to reflect emotional characteristics similar to those found among the Somatoform Disorders. Psychodynamic exploration and understanding are highly recommended, with either conjoint or concomitant counseling of the male partner since this condition involves and threatens the couple's relationship. Physical deconditioning of the vaginal musculature using graduated dilation is an effective treatment but should not be undertaken without psychotherapeutic involvement, at least to the extent of supportive counseling. Most behavioral treatment approaches are similar to those of desensitization for phobias, beginning with exposure (i.e., visual inspection and touching) and proceeding through insertion of one, then more, fingers (or lubricated graduated dilators), first by the patient herself and then by her partner. When the penis is finally used, the patient should have control of the initial speed and depth of penetration, as well as of coital position.

As with all of the experiential techniques described herein, the exercises are first described in detail (and in writing) by the clinician, and then carried out in privacy by the patient.

302.70 Atypical Psychosexual Dysfunction

Disorders similar to those described earlier but which are placed in this residual diagnostic category can usually be treated using the principles already outlined. Behavioral, "desensitization" techniques are useful, but should be undertaken by trained and experienced therapists in appropriate surroundings, with attention to the interpersonal and psychological dynamics involved. Understanding underlying pathology is especially important when the atypical dysfunction appears to involve thought disorder, major affective disorder, personality disorder, or other cardinal mental illness. Medical aspects of sexual dysfunction should not be overlooked; disorders which resemble "functional" DSM-III diagnoses but do not completely fit DSM-III criteria often involve physical illness or are iatrogenic (e.g., from medications or surgical trauma).

OTHER PSYCHOSEXUAL DISORDERS

302.00 Ego-dystonic Homosexuality

Although patients with Ego-dystonic Homosexuality, like those with Paraphilias, may come to treatment because of overt family, social, or legal problems, a significant number appear for alleviation of painful affects and inner conflicts with family or cultural mores. For some individuals, those who have been misdiagnosed or mislabeled homosexual or who painfully see themselves as homosexual because of behaviors which are insufficient to fill psychiatric criteria for homosexuality, education and brief counseling may bring significant relief. The patient may then continue his or her sexual behavior with less perceived conflict (assuming the behavior has continued up to the time of clinical evaluation), may experience a relief and strengthening of self-image which will allow entry into psychotherapy for a condition(s) other than homosexuality, or may stop feeling so badly about past "homosexual" events which are no longer taking place.

For those patients who are accurately diagnosed homosexual, and for whom this state is ego-dystonic, the treatment is far more complex and less likely to result in global alleviation of symptoms. Marks (1981b) speaks of "increasing heterosexuality" in these and in paraphilic patients, citing aversive techniques such as covert sensitization, which requires no external equipment and little participation by the therapist except for training and occasional monitoring of progress. Marks and others also discuss fading in this regard (see sections on the Paraphilias, page 158).

Socarides (1979) has written extensively on the psychoanalytic treatment of the homosexual male, including treatment of homosexual patients for symptoms which they did not identify as related to their sexual preference and patients in whom the homosexuality was so latent that the symptoms were rarely overt. Positive predictive characteristics of patients seeking analytically oriented treatment of the constellation of conflicts involved in homosexuality are similar to those which are sought in other psychotherapy patients (good premorbid adaptation, circumscribed symptoms, good ego strengths, ability to tolerate anxiety, ability to tolerate and work within the transference relationship, etc.). The empathic, understanding psychotherapist promotes the formation of the transference, which is most effectively accomplished in patients with later, rather than earlier, developmental arrest. The therapist may have to become a self-object until a true neurotic transference is achieved. As with other patients in analytically oriented treatment, attention must be paid to secondary gratifications (e.g., the "neurotic equilibrium"), which become practical barriers to eventual, lasting change.

An alternative view of the treatment of Ego-dystonic Homosexuality would address the dysphoria rather than the homosexual orientation of the patient. Thus for many therapists and patients it seems more advisable to address those matters which make the patient feel badly, leaving the homosexuality alone for the time being.

302.89   Psychosexual Disorder Not Elsewhere Classified
Conditions for which this residual diagnostic category is used should be treated with approaches which are based upon the symptoms presented and the underlying psychological, medical, or social issues which cause or influence them. Caution is again warranted in order to avoid the erroneous placing of disorders into the "psychosexual" category which upon closer examination may actually contain important features of other cardinal illness.

Chapter 12

Factitious Disorders

The treatment of the Factitious Disorders is not well established, in part because of a lack of controlled studies, the relative rarity of the disorders, and the usually unsuccessful treatment responses described in anecdotal reports.

300.16   Factitious Disorder with Psychological Symptoms
This uncommon presentation of Factitious Disorder will be discussed with the treatment of Chronic Factitious Disorder with Physical Symptoms (301.51) below. This diagnostic term is sometimes erroneously substituted for the older concept of "Ganser's Syndrome." Ganser's Syndrome, however, is clearly not under voluntary control and should be treated with a combination of environmental change (when possible—its presentation is often in prisoners), support, and temporary use of antipsychotic medication.

301.51   Chronic Factitious Disorder with Physical Symptoms
The treatment of patients with Factitious Disorder is difficult because of a lack of established approaches to which the disorder will respond, the absence of controlled studies of its treatment, and the virtual certainty that the patient will leave medical care soon after the disorder is discovered. Such measures as the blacklisting of patients and denial of hospitalization are repugnant to most physicians, and could have disastrous consequences (Hyler & Sussman, 1981). Hyler and Sussman (1981) have suggested that extensive behavior modification programs may be helpful; however, these are almost never feasible.

For those occasional patients who are successfully encouraged to pursue long-term psychotherapy, the uncovering, in a supportive surrounding, of

173

reasons for masochistic or substitutive behavior may bring marked improvement. Another area of psychotherapy may address the patient's need for attention and caring, and of anger against objects who withhold this from him. A dynamic issue which has been discussed in this context, as well as in other self-mutilating patients, has to do with an apparent need to sacrifice one part of the body (e.g., through surgery) in order to protect the whole from suicide or decompensation into psychosis.

From the above it may be inferred that treatment aimed at underlying emotional illness may be useful, particularly if the psychopathological disorder is one for which good treatments are available and which allows the patient to remain in the psychiatrist's care. For most patients, biological treatments such as psychotropic medications or ECT have not been effective in eliminating factitious physical or psychological symptoms.

Indirect assistance may be provided by the psychiatrist within a consultation or liaison setting. Communication with medical and nursing staff about the nature of the disorder and the inadvisability of punitive approaches may be helpful. The psychiatrist's input may particularly assist in decisions regarding whether or not to perform potentially hazardous procedures for diagnosis or treatment.

In either the consultation role or the individual treatment role, the psychiatrist must become the agent of the patient. The unfortunately frequent practice of a referring physician's asking the psychiatrist to be the bearer of the diagnosis undermines any future psychotherapeutic role (Hyler, 1982).

300.19　Atypical Factitious Disorder with Physical Symptoms

The treatment of patients who fall within this residual category should be based upon the presenting symptoms and underlying psychopathology, using the guidelines just described. It should be particularly noted that patients who are malingering or who have Somatoform Disorders (q.v.) should not be placed in the 300.19 category and should not be treated as if they have a Factitious Disorder.

Chapter 13

Disorders of Impulse Control
Not Elsewhere Classified

312.31   Pathological Gambling

Treatment approaches to pathological gambling often equate this disorder with addictions, particularly addiction to alcohol. The patient almost invariably presents near the end of a long, downhill course of an illness which has been destructive to himself and his family in a variety of ways. Whenever possible, treatment should employ techniques consistent with the seriousness of the patient's condition, i.e., multifaceted programs which may remove the patient from his or her environment, and/or remove the ability of the patient to further injure (usually financially) those around him or her.

Kellner (1982b) describes the highly structured residential programs available in a few centers, which initially treat the crisis in which the patient finds himself and then set out to provide an accepting milieu in which firm and consistent efforts can be made to deal with personal, family, financial, and social issues. Among the specific topics that must be addressed are those of unrealistic expectations (both positive and negative) about the treatment program. The patient may also place undue emphasis on unrealistic or non-constructive issues such as the hopelessness of getting out of debt or the belief that additional money will solve all his/her problems.

Group approaches frequently used for pathological gamblers range from private clinical settings to the broader matrix of Gamblers Anonymous. The latter now has chapters in most major cities, operating along lines similar to Alcoholics Anonymous. Family involvement at some level of the treatment should be pursued, both in terms of the long-term goals of treatment (see below) and to alleviate some of the suffering which the family is enduring.

Psychodynamic approaches to gambling generally address the obsessive, neurotic characteristics related to the winning of symbolic objects and love, challenge and mastery. Behavioral approaches, particularly aversive conditioning, are based upon the tremendous reinforcing characteristics of gambling for the patient. Although the gambling itself, by this time, is not particularly pleasurable, it has provided reinforcement on a variable ratio, variable intensity schedule which requires specialized behavioral techniques to extinguish. Neither psychodynamic nor behavioral treatment programs have proved their efficacy for patients who fill the criteria for a diagnosis of Pathological Gambling.

No matter what the approach, treatment should include attention not only to individual psychodynamics but to the patient's family environment, social and vocational situation, and debts. It must be structured so that follow-up of improvement in these categories can be maintained. The clinician should be aware of both superficial and more lasting contributors to the symptoms, such as the presence of depression and particular life stresses.

Additional therapeutic suggestions may be found in work by Wray and Dickerson (1981) and Lester (1980).

312.32   Kleptomania

The traditional treatment of Kleptomania involves psychotherapy within which underlying causes for the irresistible impulse may be discovered. In some patients, reported as cases rather than controlled studies, discovery of the psychodynamics alone is sufficient to allow behavioral change. When the onset of the disorder is not acute or associated with some identifiable event, however, reports of therapeutic success become less common and treatment outcomes rely more upon changing one's symptoms to more acceptable defense mechanisms than upon outright cure. The presence of underlying depression in many shoplifting women, not specifically diagnosed as having Kleptomania, has led to the successful use of antidepressants (notably the MAO inhibitors) in some patients (Robey, 1981).

312.33   Pyromania

The characteristics of neurotic defensive structure in Pyromania appear similar to those of Kleptomania; however, the causative psychodynamics may be quite different. The obvious danger to others of the patient's pyromanic activity dictates a need for more psychiatric or social control during treatment than is the case for Kleptomania. In inpatient settings, the safety of others must be considered paramount. The patient with this disorder is less likely than one who gambles or steals to be released on probation pending outpatient treatment.

Kellner (1982b) discusses this and other disorders of impulse control in a context of acceptance by the therapist; formation of the therapeutic relationship; exploration of the affectual, cognitive, and behavioral characteristics of pyromanic fantasies and acts; and then therapeutic intervention to change beliefs, decrease situational factors (such as tension, by desensitization), and cope with unavoidable affects (such as rage). These principles are common to the strengthening of impulse control in many patients, not only those discussed in this section on Disorders of Impulse Control. As with Kleptomania, underlying or coexisting disorders should be sought and treated.

312.34 Intermittent Explosive Disorder

This disorder may be seen as lack of modulation of anger or, perhaps in a separate group of patients, as a seizure-like condition of idiosyncratic behavior which cannot be placed as easily on a spectrum of normal to abnormal impulse control.

In the former view, that which sees the patient as having difficulty with some aspects of recognition or modulation of his or her affect (or the behavior attached to that affect, particularly of anger), treatment may focus upon these topics using biofeedback, desensitization, group therapy, and counseling which encourages careful exploration of one's behavior (such as by keeping a diary). The use of medication is controversial but generally not recommended. A few such patients may have paradoxical reactions to the benzodiazepines or alcohol, with a concomitant rage response.

Those who view this disorder, or certain patients within it, as more related to seizure phenomena (Elliott, 1978) or "episodic dyscontrol" (Monroe, 1981) recommend careful neurological workup. Anticonvulsant treatment should be considered for intractable cases, even in the absence of positive neurological findings. Carbamazepine is specifically suggested, but requires close medical follow-up because of potential adverse effects. Combinations of the more common anticonvulsants, with or without other drugs (e.g., phenytoin and thioridazine), have been tried in a number of studies. It should be noted that most research has not been with patients specifically diagnosed Intermittent Explosive Disorder but with those whose symptoms and histories were similar to those described for this diagnosis in DSM-III. Other approaches have included antidepressants and propranolol (Elliott, 1978); however, controlled studies are lacking. Propranolol appears to be more useful in those patients for whom a central nervous system trauma or lesion can be demonstrated. Lithium has been recommended for some "emotionally un-stable" patients but there is no evidence that it is consistently useful (Reid & Gutnik, 1982).

Stereotaxic surgery of various kinds has been useful in experimental ani-mals; however, its study in humans for this psychiatric (as differentiated from neurological) disorder has been severely limited.

312.35   Isolated Explosive Disorder
The nature of this diagnosis makes treatment considerations irrelevant unless there are some residual symptoms which might be medically or psychologi-cally addressed, or unless the explosive condition returns and the patient can be diagnosed Intermittent Explosive Disorder (312.34).

312.39   Atypical Impulse Control Disorder
For many clinicians, this residual category will apply to a wide variety of pa-tients. After careful differential diagnosis and ruling out of organic causes (particularly for older patients), treatment should be based upon the present-ing symptoms and underlying causes as they appear to the mental health pro-fessional. Because of the variety of treatments recommended for different im-pulse control disorders in this section (ranging from the multifaceted milieu treatment of Pathological Gambling to the anticonvulsant treatment of cer-tain Intermittent Explosive Disorders), the clinician should consider consulta-tion with and/or referral to a colleague who works often with patients of the general type being seen.

Chapter 14

Adjustment Disorder

By definition, all of these disorders are "maladaptive reactions" to identifiable stressors (American Psychiatric Association, 1980). Since the symptoms will remit or disappear once the stress is gone, or will evolve into a more permanent (effective or ineffective) coping mechanism if the stressor persists, the tasks of treatment are to deal with acute symptoms and try to promote either a return to the healthy premorbid state or an effective level of adapting to the chronic stressor. In a number of the disorders, support is important while the patient draws upon his or her own resources for improvement and growth. Support and active psychotherapeutic involvement may also prevent the patient's resolution of the adjustment disorder in a regressive, disabling manner. Treatment crises which may arise include management of suicide potential.

The psychotherapeutic approaches which work best and are most practical are usually those of crisis intervention, brief psychotherapy, counseling, and education. Brief environmental change may be helpful; however, simplistic advice such as "take a few days of vacation" is insufficient for persons who meet the criteria for these diagnoses.

Group therapy, particularly that which focuses upon enhancing self-image while showing the patient how to improve, both within a supportive environment, may be helpful. Patients with adjustment disorders often need individual attention, although it need not be intensive in nature. For those patients whose stressors continue (e.g., persons with chronic illness), a consistent group therapy environment in which transient problems can be effectively resolved may be very useful.

Pharmacotherapy of these disorders should not be emphasized. Temporary use of anxiolytic agents may be helpful; however, if the patient appears to require chronic antianxiety medication, antidepressants, or other biological treatments, then he or she should be reevaluated. This may indicate an erroneous original diagnosis or suggest that the adjustment disorder is evolving toward a chronic pattern of resolution.

While much of treatment will involve the patient alone, family members are often concerned and can benefit from reassurance, with the patient's permission, concerning the transience and treatability of the Adjustment Disorder. This is best done in a conjoint or family session soon after the initial evaluation.

309.00   Adjustment Disorder with Depressed Mood
In addition to the general principles just outlined, those patients with depressive symptoms may perceive more discomfort than other Adjustment Disorder patients, may appear more disabled, may show more symptoms of behavioral change (e.g., sleep disturbance, lack of energy), and may present with suicidal ideation and/or attempts. Unless the patient has other symptoms of Major Affective or Bipolar Disorder (in which case the Adjustment Disorder diagnosis is probably inappropriate), for example, vegetative signs or a positive dexamethasone suppression test, antidepressant medication should not be used. The antianxiety medications should be avoided as well, except perhaps short-acting preparations for sleep, since several of them can precipitate increases in the patient's dysphoria. Support and availability of the clinician, with reassurance that this experience is likely to be transient, are important for these patients. Simple, practical recommendations—not necessarily pharmacologic ones—for complaints of sleeplessness, lack of energy, and the like often have good results.

The patient should be asked about suicidal thoughts, and any suicidal ideation or behavior discussed openly. In these patients, as opposed to those with more serious depression, thoughts of suicide are more likely to be anxiety-producing and to be efforts at resolution in fantasy of real problems, than they are to be lethal. Nevertheless, the clinician must assure the patient that this topic can be discussed as any other, and that in the unlikely event that further control or treatment should be necessary it is readily available.

309.24   Adjustment Disorder with Anxious Mood
In addition to the principles outlined in the general comments above, clinical reassurance of the transience of the symptoms, and of the ability of the clinician and patient together to alleviate them, will be useful. Relaxation, medi-

tation, hypnosis, or biofeedback may be used by those therapists who prefer one or another. Temporary antianxiety medication, preferably a benzodiazepine, is often helpful. These agents provide effective control of symptoms, although (as mentioned in the section on Anxiety Disorders) they do not eliminate anxiety altogether and have no "curative" value.

309.28   Adjustment Disorder with Mixed Emotional Features
The principles outlined above address this disorder.

309.30   Adjustment Disorder with Disturbance of Conduct
In addition to the principles outlined in the general sections above, it is important for the clinician, the patient, and the patient's family to understand the differential between this disorder and other, more chronic antisocial conditions (e.g., Antisocial Personality Disorder). It may also be useful to point out that treatment of antisocial behaviors at the time of their presentation as an Adjustment Disorder will lessen the probability that the antisocial symptoms will continue as a chronic pattern of coping or adaptation once the initial stress is removed (or as the chronic stress continues).

Countertransference issues and the temptation of some therapists to take a harsh approach to persons with this disorder should be carefully monitored. In spite of the inconvenience or injury which has been caused to others, acceptance and attempts to have the patient understand that his or her symptoms are characteristics of his difficulty adjusting, and not indications of some deep inner criminality, character disorder, or evil, are very important. This approach allows the patient to see treatment as something logical and accomplishable, whose explorations and anxieties can be tolerated.

Continuing responsibility for one's actions is also in order. The therapist's acceptance of the *patient* and reassurance for his/her fragile self-image do not imply acceptance of the antisocial *acts* which place people and property in jeopardy. While the psychiatrist may support the patient in court, for example, under most circumstances these conditions should not be allowed to exonerate him or her altogether.

309.40   Adjustment Disorder with Mixed Disturbance of Emotions and Conduct
This disorder should be treated using the principles already outlined above, both at the beginning of this section and within the paragraphs on individual disorders. It should be noted that treatment for one portion of the disorder (e.g., prescription of benzodiazepines for anxiety) may have either a positive or an adverse effect on some other group of symptoms (e.g., recklessness or

self-destructive behavior). The benefits and detriments of each must be weighed. Finally, the self-destructive nature of many reckless or antisocial-appearing acts should not be overlooked.

309.23   Adjustment Disorder with Work (or Academic) Inhibition
In addition to the principles already outlined for treatment of Adjustment Disorders in general, it should be noted that disorders involving work or academic inhibition may have effects which last beyond the duration of the psychiatric symptoms themselves. In these cases, brief, supportive, goal-directed counseling (such as that found in many student health centers), while effective, may also include communication with teachers or employers. The patient can be encouraged to discuss current difficulties with the teacher or employer in person. At other times, telephone or written communication, or even having the third party attend a session if work or school is part of the stress involved, may be used. As is the case in Adjustment Disorder with Disturbance of Conduct (309.30), the issue raised should be one of specific performance and improvement of adjustment, not of responsibility for one's work or school performance. It may also be noted that work or academic inhibition implies a change in one's appearance to and involvement with peer groups and authority figures. This is true to some extent in other adjustment disorders as well, and should be addressed in counseling.

309.83   Adjustment Disorder with Withdrawal
In addition to the above general principles of treatment, the clinician should be aware that the symptom of withdrawal lends itself to isolation from sources of growth and support, and thus may increase the probability that the adjustment disorder will evolve into chronic depression or avoidance. The patient should be encouraged, perhaps by "prescription," to have a certain amount of contact with others. The family can continue at home the psychotherapist's kind but firm pressure and reassurance.

309.90   Adjustment Disorder with Atypical Features
Adjustment disorders which fall into this residual category should be treated according to the presenting symptoms, the temporary or chronic stressors involved, and the environmental and psychodynamic characteristics which are likely to have an influence upon the eventual resolution of the condition. As with other residual categories in the DSM-III, particular attention should be paid to differential diagnosis and the elimination of other cardinal mental illness from consideration.

Chapter 15

Psychological Factors Affecting Physical Condition

316.00   Psychological Factors Affecting Physical Condition
Although the psychological factors, accompanying symptoms, and treatment approaches vary widely depending upon the patient's emotional characteristics and specific physical disorder, some principles for intervention by the psychiatrist or other mental health professional, or for psychiatrically oriented approaches to be taken by the attending physician, can be enumerated. In each, the therapist should be a powerful ally of the patient. The family environment must not be neglected; formal family therapy may be important to the lasting alleviation of the disorder.

For purposes of this discussion, psychological factors affecting physical condition will be divided into three sometimes overlapping groups:

1) those in which the psychologically meaningful stimulus or process is acute, and is followed by medical complications which are acute and short-lived;

2) those in which the precipitating psychological stimulus or process is acute but the resultant medical complications are more lasting or chronic; and

3) those in which the psychological precipitating process is either ongoing or intermittent over a long period, and thus for which the medical symptoms or complications are chronic and/or recurrent.

It will be noted that the first of these (#1) is phenomenologically similar to the Adjustment Disorders discussed previously.

1) *Acute event with acute, brief reaction.* One example of such a situation might be an emotional reaction to pending surgery, which increases the probability of medical or surgical complications. Another might be an emotional reaction to isolation and threat of death while one is being treated in a medical intensive care unit. Psychiatric approaches to such conditions vary widely, depending on presentation and the individual; however, one can generally recommend a consultation-liasion approach which may suggest to treating staff careful explanation of procedures, discussion of events which occurred prior to the onset or worsening of the illness in question (Theorell, 1980), environmental changes within the hospital or other health care facility, advice to hospital staff and colleagues about communicating with the patient to allay anxieties, increasing sensory stimulation and information available (to, for example, the isolated patient), or small doses of neuroleptic or antianxiety medication, each as appropriate to the case at hand.

2) *Situations in which acute, psychologically meaningful physical or emotional stimuli or processes precipitate an ongoing medical condition or chronic worsening of medical symptoms.* Such a clinical situation may evolve from the more acute setting discussed above. Examples include some cases of psychogenic amenorrhea which begin with apparently acute stimuli and which may remit after brief psychiatric intervention (Khuri & Gehi, 1981). Some conditions may appear similar to Post-traumatic Stress Disorder (308.30, 309.81).

Treatment is often more complex than the relatively straightforward consultation-liaison or brief counseling approach frequently useful in (#1) above. The ongoing nature of the symptoms may imply greater depth of psychopathology, a more pervasive precipitating trauma, and/or more deeply embedded symptoms by the time the patient is seen by the psychiatrist. Ross et al. (1982) describe cases in which incomplete early treatment of psychologically significant stressors and the symptoms precipitated led to both medical and psychological problems in the future. The abilities of a consultation-liaison team to impact upon several levels of medical care and to follow up patients whom they have seen are important in this regard. The psychiatric approach may still be relatively brief and non-intensive, with symptom removal by a variety of means (traditional psychotherapy, biofeedback) and ongoing support frequently leading to a good resolution, especially in cases of relatively acute onset and clear-cut stressors.

3) *Patients for whom the psychologically significant event or its residua continue to influence, chronically or intermittently, the medical condition of the patient.* This group of patients includes those who fall most clearly into the classic "psychosomatic" diagnostic bailiwick. Our understanding of the psychodynamics of some of the disorders is quite specific; others have only recently been added to the seven whose developmental characteristics were brought out by Franz Alexander (1950) (ulcerative colitis, peptic ulcer, bronchial asthma, etc.).

Karasu (1979) points out that psychosomatic patients present a number of barriers to traditional psychodynamic treatment. These include the complexity of the influences between the psyche and the rest of the self, routinely profound resistance and denial, and countertransference reactions within the psychotherapist. He describes two "phases" of psychotherapy which should precede the therapeutic alliance: the "health alliance" in which the therapist has a doctor-patient relationship with the patient and is intimately involved with the medical aspects of his illness; and the "life alliance" in which as the medical condition improves the therapist begins to become a friend or teacher.

Karasu notes that these preparatory phases may last months or years before the patient becomes accessible to a more psychoanalytic approach. Bräutigam (1979) also notes the necessity for patient, lengthy treatment, perhaps including preverbal (e.g., movement, art) therapies prior to, for example, an outpatient group. Bräutigam particularly recommends group therapy and notes that shortcuts are to be avoided while one tries to narrow the discrepancy between the patient's self-image and his/her ideal. Karasu and Bräutigam both note the need for flexibility of therapeutic approach, and the lack of success of rigid psychotherapy which assumes that the psychosomatic patient will respond as a neurotic one.

Significant gains may be seen when psychotherapy is added to medical treatment. These vary with a number of factors, including the medical illness itself. For example, patients with asthma often respond well to psychotherapy aimed at altering their attitude toward the illness, whether individually or in groups. Essential hypertension, on the other hand, has shown little response to psychiatric intervention whether or not it addresses theoretical underlying, precipitating psychodynamics.

Much treatment, such as supportive therapy for a brittle diabetic, may be considered similar to the therapy of one with a chronic Adjustment Disorder to an illness. Modifying patterns of communication and relationships, altering behavioral patterns, broadening the patient's perception of external and internal situations, and use of biofeedback or other conditioning techniques may be helpful for specific goals (Cohen, 1979). These should be offered within a biopsychosocial context (Kimball, 1981). There should be a good relationship between the treating physician and the psychiatrist (Strain, 1981).

Wolpe (1980) notes that learned responses are a significant factor in most psychosomatic disorders, and discusses ways to utilize this fact in behavior therapy. An initial behavior analysis to establish a correlation between psychological factors and the somatic illness (or exacerbation thereof) is important and should be exhaustive. Following this, any of a number of techniques (systematic desensitization, flooding, biofeedback) may be effective in many patients. Asthmatics respond particularly well to desensitization of a number of types aimed at the asthmatic attack, the environment surrounding the attacks, and situations which produce key stresses.

Relaxation and other techniques have been useful for symptomatic relief of headache and hypertension; however, the effects of any behavioral approaches on the long-term treatment of hypertension are still in question. Catharsis, assertiveness training, and even simple insight have been found helpful in some psychogenic dermatologic reactions.

As noted at the beginning of this section, the author's differentiation of these syndromes is somewhat arbitrary, but may be clinically useful. The clinical characteristics are overlapping, and the principles involved in treatment of acute symptoms may apply to situations in any of the three groups.

Chapter 16

Personality Disorders

Since for the most part the existence of a Personality Disorder in and of itself does not produce discomfort, treatment is usually designed to alleviate peripheral symptoms (some of which have already been discussed), decrease social or emotional disability, or deal with some aspect of society's needs for management of, for example, the antisocial person. For some disorders, treatment is rarely an issue; for others, reliable strategies have not been developed. The depth of pathology is such that any concept of "cure" requires marked restructuring of very basic developmental characteristics. This approach has been studied for only a few of the Personality Disorders, with such attempts involving highly specialized, enormously energy-consuming therapies. Biological approaches (e.g., pharmacotherapy) may be useful for some symptoms of some disorders; however, none responds in any globally helpful fashion.

Countertransference and related feelings in the psychiatrist or psychotherapist are major issues in the treatment of the Personality Disorders. The frustration of dealing with treatment-resistant and/or primitive patients, who (unless dismissed by the therapist) may be seen over many years is obvious. Less obvious is the problem of the therapist's true countertransference, seeing in the patient frightening or distasteful aspects of one's own angry, sexual, or dependent impulses.

301.00 Paranoid Personality Disorder

Individuals with Paranoid Personality rarely come to treatment unless the disorder decompensates into one of the Axis I disorders. Those who do may do so to prove to others that "there's nothing wrong with me," or may be professional people who consult the clinician as a colleague about some problem whose source seems external to the patient. While many therapists would choose not to continue an informal, unrewarding interaction with such a person, there may be some value in allowing a benign relationship to form within which more serious problems that may arise in the future can be handled.

Pharmacotherapy is not indicated unless psychotic decompensation appears to be approaching. When the patient feels anxiety about loss of control he or she may accept, and benefit from, mild sedatives or low doses of neuroleptic medication from a physician for whom there is at least some feeling of trust. The patient should be encouraged to participate in any treatment plan that is formed, and should never be treated surreptitiously.

Patients with a Paranoid Personality may have a variety of problems with those around them, particularly with law enforcement agencies. The psychiatrist who treats patients in a legal setting should be aware of the special constraints (and occasionally advantages) of court-ordered treatment, psychiatric treatment in correctional institutions, and other aspects of having persons with this and similar personality disorders in one's caseload.

301.20   Schizoid Personality Disorder

The treatment of the condition described in DSM-III as Schizoid Personality Disorder is derived from psychotherapeutic experience, particularly relatively recent work in the understanding and restructuring of primitive developmental phenomena. Unfortunately, few such patients are able to receive and complete depth psychotherapy, even given some potential responsiveness to it. The goal of therapy described by Appel (1974) has to do with providing the patient with some sense of optimism that his or her basic needs can be met without encountering some overwhelming "collapse or suffocation." The most useful therapeutic interaction is consistent and supportive, with clear rules, an ability for the patient to set the therapeutic distance as necessary, and some tolerance for acting-out behaviors.

Medications are generally not useful except as temporary aids in cases of extraordinary anxiety. Antidepressants should not be prescribed in the absence of clinical signs of an Axis I affective disorder. Antipsychotic medication tends not to be useful for this group of patients unless signs of decompensation appear (see Schizotypal Personality Disorder, 301.22, below).

301.22   Schizotypal Personality Disorder

Schizotypal Personality Disorder involves more distortion of reality than does Schizoid Personality Disorder (301.20, above). The same psychotherapeutic principles apply; however, a need for antipsychotic medication may appear more often, and low-dose trials of high-potency neuroleptics are often indicated if the patient will accept the medication.

The various treatment considerations described later in this section for Narcissistic and Borderline Personality Disorders (301.81 and 301.83, respectively) may provide useful information for the person treating patients with Schizoid and Schizotypal Personality Disorders as well.

301.50   Histrionic Personality Disorder

Tupin (1981) notes that psychotherapy is the basic treatment for many personality disorders, including Histrionic Personality. He notes that the "good hysteric" seems to respond well to psychoanalytically oriented psychotherapy; however, the more primitive patient is more likely to respond to limited, supportive treatment. For those patients who fit the diagnosis of Histrionic Personality Disorder, the disturbance is likely to be sufficiently deep (i.e., characterologic) that intensive psychotherapy generally will not be effective.

The therapist should be aware that the reactive aspects of the disorder often lead to anxious, depressive, or other overreactions to minor emotional or external events. Techniques of brief counseling or psychotherapy within a supportive context will be needed for such responses, both in the ongoing treatment of the chronic patient and in the sporadic treatment of the histrionic patient who comes to therapy only when symptomatic. As with the other personality disorders, countertransference reactions should be expected. These may center around the demanding, self-indulgent aspects of the patient or around constantly dependent, manipulative behaviors.

Dramatic, impulsive, often poorly thought-out suicidal behavior is frequently seen. Although it may accurately be seen as manipulative or "gesture," such behavior must always be taken seriously, particularly if one is not closely familiar with a given patient. For those with whom the therapist is quite familiar, the principles of availability, consistency, and firmness outlined in the sections on the Borderline Personality may be helpful.

Medications are not indicated in the chronic treatment of Histrionic Personality. If used for brief, reactive symptoms, they should be given for only a short period, with attention to the patient's abuse potential and possible propensity for self-destructive behavior. If depressive symptoms arise, antidepressants should rarely be used in the absence of symptoms of a Major Affective Disorder. MAO inhibitors may be more successful than tricyclics. Brief deteriorations into psychosis, should they occur, can often be treated supportively or environmentally; however, low doses of high-potency neuroleptics may be considered. Such treatment should not be confused with the higher doses and extensive medication regimens reserved for the Schizophrenic and Schizophreniform Disorders.

301.81   Narcissistic Personality Disorder

Many of the treatment principles and approaches discussed for this disorder apply as well to Borderline Personality Disorder (301.83). Clinicians treating either of these conditions should be aware of the contents of both of these sections, as well as the general principles outlined throughout the portion of this book devoted to the Personality Disorders.

Most psychiatrists will, as a practical matter, treat most of their severely narcissistic patients for symptoms related to crises and relatively external Axis I diagnoses, rather than in an effort to address the personality disorder itself. As Phillips (1981) points out, symptomatic distress is often the result of some loss which has led to disrupted self-esteem via disappointment or loss of an extension of the self. Horowitz (1976) cautions the therapist to be aware of the importance of narcissism to the contiguity of the patient's psyche, to refrain from confronting the need for self-aggrandizement, and to help the patient use his or her narcissistic characteristics to reconstitute an intact self-image. Positive transference and therapeutic alliance should not be relied upon, since the patient may not be able to acknowledge the real humanness of the therapist but may have to see him/her as either superhuman or devalued.

Those patients who do not terminate treatment after symptom relief has been obtained may wish help for some of the problems related to their personality disorder, such as interpersonal difficulties or depression. Horowitz (1976) addresses this in part, offering suggestions for treatment of specific elements of the narcissistic style. Baker (1979) notes the potential for countertransference problems in which the therapist feels helpless with the narcissistic patient. He suggests that the therapist have a good understanding of the principles of the narcissistic personality style, both for interpretation to the patient and for use in combatting countertransference. Goals for ordinary psychotherapy should not be too great, since the source of these patients' difficulties lies deep in pathological development.

A number of authors have discussed group psychotherapy. Stone and Gustafson (1982) use a developmental model of anxiety and object relations which attempts to establish a working alliance. The goals are to help the patient develop a healthy individuality (rather than a resilient narcissism) so that he or she can acknowledge others as separate persons, and to decrease the need for self-defeating coping mechanisms. They feel that the first step toward developing this alliance is empathy with the surprise and hurt that the patient experiences as a result of confrontations within the group. Horwitz (1980) emphasizes the external structuring group therapy provides, which can control destructive behavior in spite of ego weakness. In groups, the therapist is less authoritative (and less threatening to the patient's grandiosity);

intensity of emotional experience is lessened; and regression is more controlled, creating a better setting for confrontation and clarification.

Outpatient analytic-expressive group therapy requires a concomitant individual relationship for most patients, which should be somewhat supportive. The need for this additional support, the likelihood of the patient's leaving the group at the first sign of psychic insult, and proneness to disorganized thinking are all found more often in the Borderline patient (q.v.). The patient with a Narcissistic Personality Disorder does not appear so vulnerable to separation anxieties as the Borderline patient, but is instead involved in issues centered around maintaining a sense of self-worth (Abler, 1980).

If the patient shows signs of good ego strength and is carefully evaluated by a psychoanalyst experienced with these disorders, then reconstruction of the personality may be undertaken. For most patients and clinicians, however, psychoanalytic work is not indicated.

The hospitalization of patients with severe Narcissistic Personality occurs frequently. For some, such as those who are quite impulsive or self-destructive, or who have poor reality-testing, this is the result of Axis I symptoms which are overlaid upon the personality disorder (see below). Hospitalizations should be brief, and the treatment specific to the particular symptom involved.

Another group of patients for whom hospitalization is indicated, provided long-term residential treatment is available, are those who have poor motivation for outpatient treatment, fragile object relationships, chronic destructive acting out, and chaotic life-styles. The inpatient program described by Hartocollis (1980) offers an intensive milieu which includes individual psychotherapy, family involvement, and a specialized residential environment. The structure is physically and emotionally secure enough to sustain the patient with severe ego weakness throughout the course of expressive, conflict-solving psychotherapy. There are small staff-patient groups within the wards, as well as large community meetings, at which feelings are shared and patients' comments taken seriously by staff. There are constructive work assignments, recreational activities, and opportunities to sublimate painfully conflictual impulses. Hartocollis notes that these make the hospital a "holding" environment rather than merely a containing one, with ultimate goals of effecting a better integrated internal world, more cohesive and modulated self-object representation, and a self-concept less vulnerable to narcissistic injury.

The individual with narcissistic and related personality disorders is likely to present with Axis I symptoms and disorders at various times in his or her life. These should be treated as described elsewhere. Caution should be observed, however, not to overdiagnose psychotic decompensation as Schizophrenia unless all DSM-III criteria are apparent. The same caveat applies to the pharmacologic treatment of depressive symptoms in the absence of clinical signs of Major Affective Disorder. When treating presenting symptoms and Axis I disorders in patients with Narcissistic Personality Disorder and other similar conditions, attention should be paid to the consequences of removing symptoms in a patient whose underlying character is primitive and/ or fragile.

301.70   Antisocial Personality Disorder

The importance of differentiation of the diagnosis of Antisocial Personality from other psychiatric diagnoses and non-illness conditions (e.g., Adult Antisocial Behavior, V71.01) cannot be overstated. Clinicians continue to treat antisocial symptoms and behaviors as if they represented the personality disorder itself, however. This approach interferes with adequate treatment planning and often leads to poor response of the patient (Reid, 1981a).

When speaking of treatment of Antisocial Personality, one is by definition speaking of adults (not children or "juvenile delinquents"). It is a truism that most characterologically antisocial persons so not actively seek therapy; however, they may come to treatment in a variety of ways, the most familiar being within a forensic setting. The traditional need for motivation in psychotherapy is not quite as important here as it is for the neurotic disorders. It may be possible for the therapist to find reasons which will keep the patient working in treatment (e.g., in order to be released from incarceration). In addition, under some circumstances the patient may begin to experience some form of dysphoria, usually either temporary anxiety about some life situation or depression. The latter may arise late in the natural course of the personality disorder, as a result of containment in a hospital or a prison in which self-stimulation is impossible, or during the course of psychotherapy itself (see below) (Reid, 1981b).

The outpatient treatment of these people is fraught with difficulty, much of which is based upon the continuing availability of ways in which the patient can escape from any exploration of his fragile core. Many of these are either seductive or frustrating for the therapist; countertransference issues are so important that intensive psychotherapists with such patients are encouraged to seek professional supervision (Lion, 1981). For those patients who do become engaged in intensive therapy, the most reliable sign of progress is the development of affect. The first affect seen is often depression, which is both surprising and uncomfortable for the patient, who is not used to experiencing such feelings. At this point the therapist should become supportive and empathic, helping the patient to understand that the discomfort is a sign of progress, that it is bearable, and that patient and therapist will work together to understand it.

Definitive inpatient treatment must be carried out on a specialized unit. There should be no patients with non-antisocial diagnoses and staff must be well experienced with this kind of patient. Carney (1978) notes the particular deficits in the truly psychopathic patient which must be addressed during the intensive residential treatment: the inability to trust, to fantasize, to feel, and to learn.

Successful inpatient programs involve long-term, strictly structured, hierarchical settings in which every aspect of the patient's life affects, and is affected by, his progress. Some, like the program at Patuxent Institute in Jessup, Maryland, control the patient's administrative status as well as other parts of his life from the day he enters the hospital. He begins with very few privileges except that of being treated as a human being. As he slowly moves through a four- or five-step hierarchy of privileges, he acquires more and more self-esteem, awareness of his emotional life, and social and interpersonal competence, leading to less need for the antisocial character style. In addition to the rigorous structure there should always be time for reflection, during which, particularly in the early stages, the patient may become "emotional" without exposing himself completely to others (although sharing one's feelings with others is a necessary later part of the treatment program).

Such inpatient/residential programs take years to complete, are moderately expensive (although far less so than ineffective incarceration), and tend to have good results, particularly if the patient receives community follow-up by the same team which treated him as an inpatient (cf., the Patuxent program). Other, generally similar programs are described elsewhere. The reader may particularly wish to consult the work of George Stürup (Stürup & Reid, 1981).

Programs for women are considerably less advanced, and tend to be much more based in correctional, rather than therapeutic issues (Benedek, 1981).

Treatment with medications has not proved helpful. Noncompliance or abuse of drugs interferes with their use for alleviation of peripheral symptoms. There is some evidence that the depression which is encountered in some patients with Antisocial Personality Disorder late in life or during intensive treatment may have endogenous features. There is no reported study of the use of antidepressants for this condition.

The family of the patient deserves education and counseling. Families are often confused by the problems which the patient either causes or encounters in spite of his superficially normal appearance (Reid, 1978). This confusion, guilt, the temptation to make restitution for the patient's criminal acts, and the frustrations of working with someone who is seen to be quite ill but who will not be treated should all be discussed openly with family members. In this regard, the author has found it helpful to suggest that they read Cleckley's *The Mask of Sanity* (1976).

301.83   Borderline Personality Disorder

Like Narcissistic Personality Disorder (q.v.), patients with Borderline Personality may be seen in a variety of settings. For the patient who comes to the clinician only during times of crisis, reality issues should rapidly be addressed in spite of the patient's frequent tendency to avoid problems (Gallahorn, 1981). Availability of local mental health facilities helps the borderline patient with occasional crisis needs to function in the community.

For those patients who can tolerate intensive psychotherapy, a process of modified psychoanalysis is generally felt to be the best long-term outpatient approach (Chessick, 1979). A few analysts, notably Kernberg (1975) and Giovacchini (1975), recommend a more classical approach. The setting of limits and the acknowledgment of the demands of reality are two important issues in psychotherapy. The patient's acting out can be dangerous for him/herself and others, and can make therapy impossible. Chessick (1979) feels that, unless limitations on behavior are observed, the treatment should not proceed and the patient should be seen as insufficiently motivated.

Transference and countertransference are particularly important aspects of psychotherapy for primitive patients such as those with Borderline or Narcissistic Personalities. The therapeutic alliance should form within the patient's real experiences with the therapist and with the treatment. The therapist must be able to tolerate repeated episodes of primitive rage, distrust, and fear. Uncovering is to be avoided in favor of bolstering of ego defenses, in order to eventually allow the patient to be less anxious about potential fragmentation and loss. The goals of therapy should be in terms of life gains toward independent functioning, and not complete restructuring of the personality. Abler (1980) notes that successful treatment of the borderline disorders may lead the patient to resemble one with a Narcissistic Personality.

Group treatment should be supportive rather than exploratory, especially in the outpatient setting. As noted in the section on the Narcissistic Personality Disorder, work in groups decreases potential discomfort related to intimacy, strong transference reactions, crises of authority, and the like.

The hospital frequently enters into the treatment of the borderline patient. Beresin and Gordon (1981) note that the emergency room can be a source of empathic reassurance, crisis intervention, and education in spite of its drawbacks for psychiatric assessment and treatment. There is no working alliance in the emergency room, so support is paramount and interpretation should be absent. Medications should be directed at specific symptoms or at crisis management. Disposition is difficult, with power struggles often being part of the negotiations. Immediate return to the ongoing outpatient therapeutic system is important, as is referral for new psychotherapeutic treatment if the patient has no therapist. The clinician must be careful not to reinforce the splitting which may be present in a patient who is already being treated elsewhere but turns also to the emergency room.

Other clinicians feel that hospitalization can be an important part of the long-term improvement of the patient. Nurnberg and Suh (1982) note that short-term inpatient treatment should direct the patient toward responsible actions and assist in transition to definitive outpatient therapy. Marcus (1981) recommends the use of acute hospitalization early in the treatment of borderline patients (although Marcus does not specify a DSM-III diagnosis of Borderline Personality Disorder). Acute hospitalization may allow for more accurate diagnosis and observation of the defensive organization of the patient. In addition, during the hospitalization period the patient's environmental and interpersonal supportive systems can be evaluated in preparation for the outpatient tasks to come.

The issue of the hospital's potentiating the tremendous regressive potential in these patients must be addressed. There should be a dependable situation on the ward, not a dependent one (Peteet & Gutheil, 1979). Hospital units which provide long-term treatment for borderline patients should be highly specialized, and should not confuse the major psychodynamic issues involved with those more typical of frankly psychotic, severely depressed, or neurotic patients.

A number of authors feel that the borderline patient with high regressive potential can best be treated in a long-term, intensive, highly structured inpatient environment. The characteristics of this environment and the treatment within it are much the same as those described in the section on Narcissistic Personality Disorder (q.v.).

Sadivoy et al. (1979) note possible negative responses of the borderline patient to intensive inpatient treatment, which may be due to overstimulation of the emotional abilities of these patients. Unless the treatment environment is highly structured and the staff are sensitive to the needs and deficits of the patient, transient psychosis may be encountered. Closeness with the patient should be developed gradually, to allow him or her to experience, and then contain and work with, feelings of panic. Goals include decreasing acting out, clearly identifying and working with inappropriate behaviors and feelings, accepting with the patient the magnitude of the therapeutic task, fostering more effective interpersonal relationships, and working with both real and transference relationships within the hospital. The long-term treatment program should be seen as an environment in which the patient experiences development, and in which staff (particularly the primary therapist)ʼconsistently accompany and empathize with the patient (Chessick, 1982).

The rapid mood shifts in Borderline Personality patients make suicidal behavior common and dangerous. Suicide potential should be particularly carefully evaluated in the presence of poor reality-testing or incipient psychosis.

The use of medications in the treatment of borderline patients is a complex topic. There is no drug of choice, and many clinicians feel that avoidance of medications is important in both the short- and long-run. It is, however, clear that low doses of high potency neuroleptics (e.g., haloperidol) may be helpful for disorganized thinking and some psychotic symptoms. Depression is also often amenable to drug treatment, either with an antidepressant (especially if criteria for Major Affective Disorder are present) or, in some cases, with neuroleptics. The latter are particularly recommended for the psychotic symptoms mentioned above, and for patients who show anger which must be controlled (Leone, 1982; Lyskowski & Psuang, 1980). Dosages should generally be low and the medication should never be given without adequate psychosocial intervention. The repeated use of medication for patients' frequent complaints of anxiety should be considered only with caution.

Treatment of other symptoms and Axis I disorders which occasionally present in these patients should be as outlined elsewhere in this volume; however, the underlying personality disorder must not be ignored. These patients are fragile and prone to rapid disorganization or deterioration.

301.82　Avoidant Personality Disorder

The treatment of the patient with Avoidant Personality Disorder should take into consideration the similarities of this disorder with many of the others discussed herein, but should also consider important differences between, for example, the Avoidant patient and the Schizoid (who possesses a deficit in relating ability rather than a defense against relating) or the Borderline Personality (which reflects a more severe and dysfunctional personality syndrome) (Millon, 1981).

For those patients who come to treatment, the issue of the "neurotic equilibrium" which would be upset by any change in symptoms must be addressed from the beginning. Initial supportive treatment and enhanced self-image may allow some tentative exploration—within the safety of the therapeutic relationship—of interactions with others and with the environment. Although there are no research reports of treatment of this disorder (which is newly defined in DSM-III), group therapy with a carefully selected group of patients would seem to offer opportunities to explore growth within a protected setting. Specific treatments for particular symptoms of Axis I disorders such as anxiety or phobia might be considered.

301.60 Dependent Personality Disorder

As with many of the other personality disorders, patients with this diagnosis are unlikely to seek treatment. They may, however, wish to explore reasons for lack of social or vocational success, and may suffer considerable loss when an important figure leaves them in one way or another. Referrals of dependent patients within a consultation-liaison framework are common; however, many of these patients' characteristics are related to their medical illness or the hospital setting, and do not fill DSM-III criteria.

The primary therapeutic modality for personality disorders such as this is psychotherapy. An important early therapeutic task is acceptance by the therapist of much of the same dependence that the patient feels toward others in his or her life. The symptoms and psychodynamics can then be discussed firsthand, rather than in the patient's reports of feelings about others. The therapist's support of the patient's individuation from others (and now from the therapist as well) should include practical issues such as jobs and housing. Anxiety and depression may result, and should be taken seriously since severely dependent patients may harbor a potential for overwhelming despondency or rage against the self or others (Kiev, 1976). Situations of severe loss or intense affect in these patients should lead the therapist to consider protective measures such as hospitalization, in which the patient can be contained to some extent and definitive therapy for Axis I symptoms carried out in a controlled setting.

Patients with this condition tend to improve with supportive, insight-oriented individual or group therapy. Termination is a delicate task, and should be a joint decision. The therapist should be flexible, allowing the patient to return as needed (Malinow, 1981).

301.40 Compulsive Personality Disorder

Patients with Compulsive Personality Disorder who seek treatment usually do so because of symptoms which reflect, or are similar to, Axis I diagnoses of Obsessive Compulsive Disorder, Affective Disorder, or occasionally Paranoia. The treatment of the personality disorder itself should be psychotherapeutic, and may be intensive in nature if the patient is sufficiently motivated and tolerant. Needs to control and related fears of destructive impulses are important issues at all levels of treatment, from simple scheduling requests, to intellectualization and rationalization, to other resistances to fantasy and free association. Many of the characteristics which lead to a successful life for such a patient, and which appear to the inexperienced therapist to make for an excellent therapeutic candidate, are actually symptoms which can become serious impediments to psychotherapy (Tarachow, 1963).

The therapist must avoid competing with the patient and should be able to tolerate the patient's verbal attacks, retaining a therapeutic posture rather than allowing the session to deteriorate into an intellectual discussion or otherwise nonproductive interchange. Those patients with Compulsive Personality Disorder who show signs of deteriorating toward severe rituals or paranoia under stress should probably not be treated so intensively.

The use of medications in these patients is generally not productive. Although many will have read a psychiatry text and may request a specific drug (which they are, incidentally, not likely to abuse), medication considerations should be limited to those already mentioned in the discussions on Obsessive Compulsive Disorder (page 145), Paranoia (page 124) and severe depression.

301.84   Passive-Aggressive Personality Disorder

Treatment of these patients is similar to, but less rewarding than, the treatment of the patient with a Dependent Personality (q.v.). Psychotherapy is likely to be frustrating; however, the fact that the passive-aggressive symptoms often severely interfere with work or social goals may allow the patient to participate long enough to form a therapeutic alliance. Clear rules of therapy must be outlined; those which involve schedules, billing, and the like should be provided in writing so that patient and therapist do not spend inordinate amounts of time arguing over something which the patient calls forgetfulness, but the therapist calls (sometimes pejoratively) resistance.

Beneath the passive-aggressive symptoms lie not only anxiety about what might be found in treatment but also a potential for severe depression. Trapping the patient in a therapeutic bind, or the presence of an environmental situation which cannot be escaped through the usual passive-aggressive means, can lead to an escalation of defensive behavior, including suicide. Some clinicians suggest therapy with antidepressants at this point; however, caution should be exercised in prescribing and hospitalization may be required.

As with many of the personality disorders, countertransference and related issues must be carefully considered. One commonly hears the term "passive-aggressive" used to connote manipulative or frustrating patients with punishing, derisive, or other nonprofessional inflections. Although a therapist may feel angry, he or she should remember that the patient's behavior, even if apparently voluntary, is defending against severe anxiety or deterioration.

301.89   Atypical, Mixed or Other Personality Disorder

Patients who qualify for these residual personality disorder diagnoses should be treated based upon the clinician's estimation of personality dynamics, presenting symptoms, and interactions among them.

Chapter 17

V Codes for Conditions Not Attributable to a Mental Disorder That Are a Focus of Attention or Treatment

V65.20   Malingering
Since by definition there is no primary illness to treat once malingering has been established, there remain only a couple of issues of management of the patient who is felt to be voluntarily misrepresenting his symptoms for some conscious reason (e.g., to obtain money or avoid some sort of work). The most obvious of these is an offer of understanding and counsel to the person who feels that he or she must use this dishonest course of action. Sometimes education with respect to social agencies which are available to help with financial problems, the possible consequences of one's dishonesty, or even the fact that faking an illness really is dishonest and a serious misuse of resources may be beneficial.

The clinician's temptation to tell someone about the malingering should be contained. In addition to the possibility that the diagnosis may be in error, this author would disagree with Getto (1982) that one of the treatment goals is to make the malingering diagnosis available to legal, health, and social agencies with which the patient may have contact. The physician who does this runs considerable risk of breach of ethics and could under some circumstances be liable for slander or libel (unless he or she has been retained by an agency to determine what illness, if any, is present, such as in the case of a Social Security disability evaluation). It seems more prudent, if less gratifying, to note in the record that one is unable to find any medical or psychiatric basis for the individual's complaints.

V62.89   Borderline Intellectual Functioning

This category, which comprises the majority of retarded individuals, really represents a borderline level of mental retardation (Strider & Menolascino, 1981). For the most part, these people have few serious difficulties in society; however, they may be prone to problems in those areas in which one's cognitive abilities or fund of knowledge are important for coping with personal or environmental problems. Supportive treatment, along with relevant education for the patient when such problems or crises develop, is almost always helpful. One may wish to counsel the family of the individual as well, and be sure that the patient knows of available help from social agencies (for example, employment counseling for a worker who has lost his job).

Much of the frustration of the person with Borderline Intellectual Functioning is related to how he or she is treated by an uneducated or prejudiced public. Education of the family and community and/or discussions with school or work officials may be helpful. When problems are more troublesome, as in the case of the person with a conduct disorder, flexible, practical therapeutic measures should be employed rather than traditional approaches such as individual or group psychotherapy.

Institutionalization or other infantilizing procedures are never necessary for the treatment of Borderline Intellectual Functioning per se.

V71.01   Adult Antisocial Behavior

Repeated antisocial behavior which is not due to one of the mental disorders already discussed (including a reactive Adjustment Disorder) can be treated with a variety of approaches; however, considerable effort is required for the design, community acceptance, implementation, and ongoing operation of treatment programs. Individual and group psychotherapy alone have poor records of success, as do all of the biological therapies, ordinary psychiatric hospitalization, or simple incarceration. Inpatient hospitalization at institutions such as those discussed for criminals with Antisocial Personality (page 192) may be successful for some patients; however, the majority of persons with Adult Antisocial Behavior do not commit crimes sufficient to allow their being sentenced to several years of maximum security treatment.

Two relatively short-term treatment approaches have met with some success and are extremely cost-effective. The first is represented by several different, highly specialized community-based offender programs (Reid &

Solomon, 1981). In these, an offender (usually a young adult) is accepted into a highly structured local residential setting. His passage through a hierarchy of carefully chosen privileges and responsibilities is supervised by experienced counselors and peers. Such programs are practical and multifaceted, stress individual and group responsibility (often including work and restitution), and generally last a minimum of five-to-six months.

The second treatment approach which has had notable success is that of the so-called "wilderness program" (Reid & Matthews, 1980). Such programs, exemplified by those of Matthews and Kimball in New Mexico, last two-to-three weeks. Offenders (court-diverted or nearing parole) spend time isolated with peers and counselors in a wilderness environment which is at once highly stressful and not "connable." Individual and group responsibility is imperative, sometimes even necessary for survival. The experience is not merely one of physical endurance, but is combined with specialized counseling in an effort to integrate the individual's daily experiences and responses with his emotional deficits (such as low self-image, absence of social skills, and lack of confidence beneath a veneer of antisocial bravado). The wilderness program is not seen as an end in itself but as one part of a broader, individualized treatment plan which extends into the community to which the offender will eventually go.

Recidivism rates for both the wilderness and the community residential programs described above are much better than those for any other form of treatment. Follow-up studies of wilderness program participants, for example, indicate fairly stable positive changes in self-image, social ability, problem-solving, confidence, and social independence (Cytrynbaum & Ken, 1975; Kimball, 1979; Walsh & Golins, 1976).

V71.02   Childhood or Adolescent Antisocial Behavior

The treatment of many of these behaviors is discussed in Chapter 1 on Disorders Usually First Evident in Infancy, Childhood or Adolescence. It is important that children or adolescents not be given this diagnosis if their antisocial behavior forms a pattern which can be diagnosed elsewhere in the DSM-III. It is equally important that persons under the age of about 21 not be given a diagnosis of Antisocial Personality under any circumstances. Those who wish an extensive reference on the treatment of childhood antisocial syndromes may wish to consult work by Morrison (1981).

V62.30   Academic Problem

Treatment of this disorder in the absence of any other diagnosable mental disorder should be based upon simple counseling within a context of exploration of possible family or environmental stresses. As with many of the other V

Code conditions, one should be aware of the dangers of overdiagnosis and mislabeling of conditions not attributable to a mental disorder.

V62.20   Occupational Problem
The same basic treatment principles apply as are mentioned above under Academic Problem (V62.30).

V62.82   Uncomplicated Bereavement
Although the psychiatrist (or more frequently the family physician) may be consulted about some of the more striking symptoms of normal grief, one pitfall of treatment is overdiagnosis. The patient should not be told, or treated as if, he or she has an aberrant grief reaction or a serious depression unless he or she does not qualify for this V Code condition. Support and guidance may be given, however, with reassurance that the feelings are normal and should not be avoided. The therapist should show approval of the many feelings experienced by the grieving person, including anger toward the lost object. Counseling to the individual and to well-meaning family or friends should include a caveat against overprotection. That is, such activities as attending funeral and memorial services, returning to the home where the deceased lived, and putting away his or her possessions (and, with them, memories) should be encouraged as imperative for grieving individuals of all ages. The clinician should make it clear that he or she is available, but need not be intrusive.

If the grief remains unresolved for a particularly long time, with persistent yearning, overidentification with the deceased, and/or inability to express sadness or rage (Melges & DeMaso, 1980), then Uncomplicated Bereavement may no longer be an appropriate diagnosis and some sort of grief-resolution therapy should be offered. This may include helping the patient to make a decision to grieve, using techniques of guided imagery or guided mourning (Mawson et al., 1981), and assistance in constructing a life and an identity in the absence of the lost object.

V15.81   Noncompliance with Medical Treatment
Noncompliance in the absence of any of the mental disorders already discussed may be treated with education (about one's illness or the treatment involved) or counseling (e.g., concerning the pros and cons of religious proscriptions against blood transfusions). Counseling with family members or with frustrated medical staff who are having difficulty accepting the patient's decision may be indirectly helpful, for example by easing the tension between nursing staff and patient which can adversely affect other aspects of patient care.

V62.89   Phase of Life Problem or Other Life Circumstance Problem

The tremendous variety of problems which might fall into this category is too broad to address completely. The educational and counseling principles already discussed should suffice for most cases. The therapist should be alert for countertransference and related issues; for example, those of a young therapist treating an older patient with concerns about retirement, or a therapist with particular values who attempts to give objective counseling to a patient with opposing views.

V61.10   Marital Problem

In the absence of other mental disorder, including Adjustment Disorder, the goals of the therapist are generally to provide information and counseling, be an objective observer, recognize problems in communication and facilitate their resolution, and the like. To some extent, the therapist may wish to become a negotiator; however, most authors recommend against placing oneself in the position of "referee."

The question of whether a therapist should assist with the completion of a separation or divorce, when he or she feels that it is appropriate or inevitable, may occur. This author would recommend that the therapist be certain that such decisions are made by one or both members of the couple and not by the therapist.

Although patients may describe symptoms which make diagnosis of Axis I disorders tempting, marital problems in their normal course should be followed without overdiagnosis or overtreatment.

V61.20   Parent-Child Problem

The general principles of counseling in parent-child problems are occasionally similar to those of marital problems; however, practical issues, psychodynamics, and the fact that one member of the parent-child dyad is a child make specific issues quite different. The variety of potential conflicts and problems which may arise and the intricacy of family therapies involved make complete discussion impossible in this volume. For further discussion of some of the principles of treatment of children within their families, the reader is referred to the section on Disorders First Evident in Infancy, Childhood, or Adolescence. For a comprehensive discussion of evaluation and treatment of children within their family contexts, the clinician may wish to consult work by French (1977).

V61.80   Other Specified Family Circumstances

These conditions should be addressed according to the presenting complaints and situations as perceived by the clinician. The same general principles of education, counseling, and avoidance of overdiagnosis apply.

V61.81 Other Interpersonal Problem

These conditions should be addressed according to the presenting complaints and situations as perceived by the clinician. The same general principles of education, counseling, and avoidance of overdiagnosis apply.

References

Abler, G.: A treatment framework for adult patients with borderline and narcissistic personality disorders. *Bulletin of the Menninger Clinic,* 44(2):171–180, 1980.

Alexander, F. G.: *Psychosomatic Medicine: Its Principles and Applications.* New York: Norton, 1950.

American Psychiatric Association Task Force on Nomenclature and Statistics: *Diagnostic and Statistical Manual of Mental Disorders, Third Edition.* Washington, D.C.: American Psychiatric Association, 1980.

Andrews, G., and Harvey, R.: Does psychotherapy benefit neurotic patients? A reanalysis of the Smith, Glass, and Miller data. *Archives of General Psychiatry,* 38:1203–1208, 1981.

Appel, G.: An approach to the treatment of schizoid phenomena. *Psychoanalytic Review,* 61:99–113, 1974.

Arieti, S.: Psychotherapy of schizophrenia: New or revised procedures. *American Journal of Psychotherapy,* 34(4):464–476, 1980.

Baker, H. S.: The conquering hero quits: Narcissistic factors in underachievement and failure. *American Journal of Psychotherapy,* 33(3):418–427, 1979.

Bastani, J. B., and Kentsmith, D. K.: Psychotherapy with wives of sexual deviants. *American Journal of Psychotherapy,* 34(1):20–25, 1980.

Benedek, E. P.: Treatment of the female offender: One facility's experience. In W. H. Reid (Ed.), *The Treatment of Antisocial Syndromes.* New York: Van Nostrand Reinhold, 1981.

Benson, D. F., Stuss, D. T., Naeser, M. A., Weir, W. S., Kaplan, E. F., and Levine, H. L.: The long-term effects of prefrontal leukotomy. *Archives of Neurology,* 38:165–169, 1981.

Beresin, E., and Gordon, C.: Emergency ward management of the borderline patient. *General Hospital Psychiatry,* 3:237–244, 1981.

Berlin, F. S., and Meinecke, C. F.: Treatment of sex offenders with antiandrogenic medication: Conceptualization, review of treatment modalities, and preliminary findings. *American Journal of Psychiatry,* 138(5):601–607, 1981.

Blackburn, I. M., Bishop, S., Glen, A. I. M., Whalley, L. J., and Christie, J. E.: The efficacy of cognitive therapy in depression: A treatment trial using cognitive therapy and pharmacotherapy, each alone and in combination. *British Journal of Psychiatry,* 139:181–189, 1981.

Blair, C. D., and Lanyon, R. I.: Exhibitionism: Etiology and treatment. *Psychological Bulletin,* 89(3):439–463, 1981.

Bowers, M. K.: Therapy of multiple personality. *International Journal of Clinical and Experimental Hypnosis,* 19:57–65, 1971.

Bradford, J.: Personal communication, 1982.

Branchy, M. H., Branchy, L. B., and Richardson, M. A.: Effects of neuroleptic adjustment on clinical condition and tardive kinesia in schizophrenic patients. *American Journal of Psychiatry*, 138:608–612, 1981.

Bräutigam, W.: Aspects of therapy in psychosomatic medicine. *Psychotherapy and Psychosomatics*, 32:41–51, 1979.

Carney, F.: Inpatient treatment programs. In W. H. Reid (Ed.), *The Psychopath: A Comprehensive Study of Antisocial Disorders and Behaviors*. New York: Brunner/Mazel, 1978.

Chessick, R. D.: A practical approach to the psychotherapy of the borderline patient. *American Journal of Psychotherapy*, 33(4):531–546, 1979.

Chessick, R. D.: Intensive psychotherapy of a borderline patient. *Archives of General Psychiatry*, 39:413–419, 1982.

Cleckley, H.: *The Mask of Sanity*, 5th Edition. St. Louis: C. V. Mosby, 1976.

Cohen, S. I.: Updating the model for psychosomatic problems. *Psychotherapy and Psychosomatics*, 32:72–90, 1979.

Cooper, A. J.: Short-term treatment in sexual dysfunction: A review. *Comprehensive Psychiatry*, 22(2):206–217, 1981.

Coppen, A., Abou-Saleh, M. T., Milln, P., Bailey, J., Metcalfe, M., Burns, B. H., and Armond, A.: Lithium continuation therapy following electroconvulsive therapy. *British Journal of Psychiatry*, 139:284–287, 1981.

Cytrynbaum, S., and Ken, K.: *The Connecticut Wilderness Program: A Preliminary Report*. State of Connecticut, Counsel on Human Services, Hartford, Connecticut, 1975.

Davidson, J. R. T., Miller, R. D., Turnbull, C. D., and Sullivan, J. L.: Atypical depression. *Archives of General Psychiatry*, 39:527–534, 1982.

Donlon, P. T., Hopkin, J. T., Tupin, J. P., Wicks, J. J., Wahba, M., and Meadow, A.: Haloperidol for acute schizophrenic patients. An evaluation of three oral regimens. *Archives of General Psychiatry*, 37(6):691–695, 1980.

Elliott, F. A.: Neurological aspects of antisocial behavior. In W. H. Reid (Ed.), *The Psychopath: A Comprehensive Study of Antisocial Disorders and Behaviors*. New York: Brunner/Mazel, 1978.

Fogelson, D. L., Marder, S. R., and Van Putten, T.: Dialysis for schizophrenia: Review of clinical trials and implications for further research. *American Journal of Psychiatry*, 137(5):605–607, 1980.

French, A. P.: *Disturbed Children and Their Families*. New York: Human Sciences Press, 1977.

Freund, K.: Therapeutic sex drive reduction. *Acta Psychiatrica Scandinavica*, 62(Supp. 287):1–38, 1980.

Gagné, P.: Treatment of sex offenders with medroxyprogesterone acetate. *American Journal of Psychiatry*, 138(5):644–646, 1981.

Gallahorn, G. E.: Borderline personality disorders. In J. R. Lion (Ed.), *Personality Disorders: Diagnosis and Management*, 2nd Edition. Baltimore: Williams and Wilkins, 1981.

Getto, C. J.: V codes for conditions not attributable to a mental disorder that are a focus of treatment. In J. H. Greist, J. W. Jefferson, and R. L, Spitzer (Eds.), *Treatment of Mental Disorders*. New York: Oxford University Press, 1982.

Getto, C. J., and Ochitill, H.: Psychogenic pain disorder. In J. H. Griest, J. W. Jefferson, and R. L. Spitzer (Eds.), *Treatment of Mental Disorders*. New York: Oxford University Press, 1982.

Giovacchini, P.: *Psychoanalysis of Character Disorders*. New York: Jason Aronson, 1975.

Goldberg, H. L., Rickels, K., and Finnerty, R.: Treatment of neurotic depression with a new antidepressant. *Journal of Clinical Psychopharmacology*, 1(6 Supp.):35S–38S, 1981.

Gorman, J. M., Fyer, A. F., Gliklich, J., King, D., and Klein, D. F.: Effect of imipramine on prolapsed mitral valves of patients with panic disorder. *American Journal of Psychiatry*, 138(7):977–978, 1981.

Graber, B. G.: *Circumvaginal Musculature and Sexual Function*. Basel, Switzerland: S. Karger, 1982.

Graber, B. G.: Demystifying "sex therapy." *American Journal of Psychotherapy*, 35(4):481–488, 1981.

Green, R.: Gender identity disorders and transvestism. In J. H. Griest, J. W. Jefferson, and R. L. Spitzer (Eds.), *Treatment of Mental Disorders*. New York: Oxford University Press, 1982.

Hartocollis, P.: Long-term hospital treatment for adult patients with borderline and narcissistic disorders. *Bulletin of the Menninger Clinic*, 44(2):212–226, 1980.

Herrmann, W. M., and Beach, R. C.: Pharmacotherapy for sexual offenders: Review of the actions of antiandrogens with special references to their psychic effect. *Modern Problems in Pharmacopsychiatry*, 15:182–194, 1980.

Hoehn-Saric, R., Merchant, A. F., Keyser, M. L., and Smith, V. K.: Effects of clonidine on anxiety disorders. *Archives of General Psychiatry*, 38:1278–1282, 1981.

Horowitz, M.: *Stress Response Syndromes*. New York: Jason Aronson, 1976.

Horwitz, L.: Group psychotherapy for borderline and narcissistic patients. *Bulletin of the Menninger Clinic*, 44(2):181–200, 1980.

Hyler, S. E.: Factitious illness. *Audio Digest Psychiatry*, 11(2), January, 1982.

Hyler, S. E., and Sussman, N.: Chronic factitious disorder with physical symptoms (the Munchausen Syndrome). *Psychiatric Clinics of North America*, 4(2):365–377, 1981.

Insel, T. R.: Obsessive compulsive disorder—Five clinical questions and a suggested approach. *Comprehensive Psychiatry*, 23(3):241–251, 1982.

International Drug Therapy Newsletter. New hope for tricyclic refractory unipolar depressives? 16(7):25–27, 1981a.

International Drug Therapy Newsletter. Alprazolam: A new benzodiazepine anxiolytic. 16(10):37–40, 1981b.

Kaplan, H. S.: *The New Sex Therapy*. New York: Brunner/Mazel, 1974.

Kaplan, H. S.: *Disorders of Sexual Desire*. New York: Brunner/Mazel, 1979.

Karasu, T. B.: Psychotherapy of the psychosomatic patient. *American Journal of Psychotherapy*, 33(3):354–364, 1979.

Keller, A. C., Althof, S. E., and Lothstein, L. M.: Group therapy with gender-identity patients — A four year study. *American Journal of Psychotherapy*, 36(2):223–228, 1982.

Kellner, R.: Psychotherapy in psychosomatic disorders: A survey of controlled studies. *Archives of General Psychiatry* 32:1021–1030, 1975.

Kellner, R.: Psychotherapeutic strategies in hypochondriasis: A clinical study. *American Journal of Psychotherapy*, 36(2):146–156, 1982a.

Kellner, R.: Disorders of impulse control. In J. H. Greist, J. W. Jefferson, and R. L. Spitzer (Eds.), *Treatment of Mental Disorders*. New York: Oxford University Press, 1982b.

Kentsmith, D. K., and Eaton, M. T.: *Treating Sexual Problems in Medical Practice*. New York: Arco Publishing, 1979.

Kernberg, O.: *Borderline Conditions and Pathological Narcissism*. New York: Jason Aronson, 1975.

Khuri, R., and Gehi, M.: Psychogenic amenorrhea: An integrative review. *Psychosomatics*, 22(10):883–893, 1981.

Kiev, A.: Cluster analysis profiles of suicide attempts. *American Journal of Psychiatry*, 133(2):150–153, 1976.

Kimball, C. P.: *The Biopsychosocial Approach to the Patient*. Baltimore: Williams and Wilkins, 1981.

Kimball, R. O.: *Wilderness Experience Program: Final Evaluation Report*. Santa Fe, NM, Health and Environment Department, 1979.

Lazare, A.: Conversion symptoms. *New England Journal of Medicine*, 305(13):745–748, 1981.

Lehmann, C. R., Ereshefsky, L., Saklad, S. R., and Mings, T. E.: Very high dose loxapine in refractory schizophrenic patients. *American Journal of Psychiatry*, 138:1212–1214, 1981.

Leone, N. F.: Response of borderine patients to loxapine and chlorpromazine. *Journal of Clinical Psychiatry*, 43(4):148–150, 1982.

Lester, D.: The treatment of compulsive gambling. *International Journal of the Addictions*, 15(2):201–206, 1980.

Lewis, J. L., and Winokur, G.: The induction of mania: A natural history study with controls. *Archives of General Psychiatry*, 39:303–306, 1982.

Liberman, R. P., and Eckman, T.: Behavior therapy vs insight-oriented therapy for repeated suicide attemptors. *Archives of General Psychiatry*, 38:1126–1130, 1981.

Liebowitz, M. R., and Klein, D. F.: Differential diagnosis and treatment of panic attacks and phobic states. *Annual Review of Medicine*, 32:583–599, 1981.

Linden, W.: Exposure treatments for focal phobias: A review. *Archives of General Psychiatry*, 38:769–775, 1981.

Lion, J. R.: Countertransference and other psychotherapy issues. In W. H. Reid (Ed.), *The Treatment of Antisocial Syndromes*. New York: Van Nostrand Reinhold, 1981.

Lothstein, L. M.: Sex reassignment surgery: Historical, bioethical, and theoretical issues. *American Journal of Psychiatry*, 139(4):417–426, 1982.

Lyskowski, J. C., and Psuang, M. T.: Precautions in treating DSM-III borderline personality disorder. *American Journal of Psychiatry*, 137(1):100–112, 1980.

Malinow, K. L.: Dependent personality. In J. R. Lion (Ed.), *Personality Disorders: Diagnosis and Management*, 2nd Edition. Baltimore: Williams and Wilkins, 1981.

Marcus, E.: Use of the acute hospital unit in the early phase of long-term treatment of borderline psychotic patients. *Psychiatric Clinics of North America*, 4:133–144, 1981.

Marks, I. M.: *Living with Fear*. New York: McGraw-Hill, 1978a.

Marks, I. M.: Behavioral psychotherapy of adult neurosis. In S. Garfield and A. E. Bergin (Eds.), *Handbook of Psychotherapy and Behavioral Modification*, 2nd Edition. New York: Wiley, 1978b.

Marks, I. M.: Review of behavioral psychotherapy, I: Obsessive-compulsive disorders. *American Journal of Psychiatry*, 138(5):584–592, 1981a.

Marks, I. M.: Review of behavioral psychotherapy, II: Sexual disorders. *American Journal of Psychiatry*, 138(6):750–756, 1981b.

Marks, I. M., Stern, R. S., Mawson, D., Cobb, J. P., and McDonald, R.: Clomipramine and exposure for obsessive-compulsive rituals. *British Journal of Psychiatry*, 136:1–25, 1980.

Marmor, J.: The psychodynamic approach the the treatment of sexual problems. In M. R. Zales (Ed.), *Eating, Sleeping, and Sexuality: Treatment of Disorders in Basic Life Functions*. New York: Brunner/Mazel, 1982.

Masters, W., and Johnson, V.: *Human Sexual Inadequacy*. Boston: Little, Brown and Company, 1970.

Mawson, D., Marks, I., Ramm, E., and Stern, R.: Guided mourning for morbid grief: A controlled study. *British Journal of Psychiatry*, 138:185–193, 1981.

May, P. R. A., Tuma, A. H., and Dixon, W. J.: Schizophrenia: A follow-up study of the results of five forms of treatment. *Archives of General Psychiatry*, 38:776–784, 1981.

May, P. R. A., Van Putten, T., Jenden, D. J., Yale, C., and Dixon, W. J.: Chlorpromazine levels and the outcome of treatment in schizophrenic patients. *Archives of General Psychiatry*, 38:202–207, 1981.

McCreadie, R., Mackie, M., Morrison, D., and Kidd, J.: Once weekly pimozide versus fluphenazine decanoate and maintenance therapy in chronic schizophrenia. *British Journal of Psychiatry*, 140:280–286, 1982.

Melges, F. T. and DeMaso, D. R.: Grief-resolution therapy: Reliving, revising, and revisiting. *American Journal of Psychotherapy*, 34(1):51–60, 1980.

Menuck, M., and Voineskos, G.: Rapid parenteral treatment of acute psychosis. *Comprehensive Psychiatry*, 22(4):351–361, 1981.

Millon, T.: The avoidant personality. In J. R. Lion (Ed.), *Personality Disorders: Diagnosis and Management*, 2nd Edition. Baltimore: Williams and Wilkins, 1981.

Minchiello, W.: Behavior therapy of obsessive-compulsive disorders. *Practical Reviews in Psychiatry* (audio tape), 6(9), 1981.

Monroe, R. R.: The problem of impulsivity in personality disturbances. In J. R. Lion (Ed.), *Personality Disorders: Diagnosis and Management*, 2nd edition. Baltimore: Williams and Wilkins, 1981.

Morrison, H. L.: The asocial child: Perspectives on treatment. In W. H. Reid (Ed.), *The Treatment of Antisocial Syndromes*. New York: Van Nostrand Reinhold, 1981.

Mosher, L. R., and Keith, S. J.: Research on the psychosocial treatment of schizophrenia: A summary report. *American Journal of Psychiatry*, 137(5):623–631, 1979.

Munby, M., and Johnston, D. W.: Agoraphobia: The long-term follow-up of behavioral treatment. *British Journal of Psychiatry*, 137:418–427, 1980.

Murphy, M. F., and Davis, K. L.: Biological perspectives in chronic pain, depression, and organic mental disorders. *Psychiatric Clinics of North America*, 4(2):223–237, 1981.

Mutter, C. B.: A hypnotherapeutic approach to exhibitionism: Outpatient therapeutic strategy. *Journal of Forensic Sciences*, 26:129–133, 1981.

Neborsky, R., Janowsky, D., Munson, E., and Depry, D.: Rapid treatment of acute psychotic symptoms with high- and low-dose haloperidol: Behavioral considerations. *Archives of General Psychiatry*, 38:195–199, 1981.

Neborsky, R., Janowsky, D., Munson, E., Hornbeck, C., and Depry, D.: Behavioral prediction of response to haloperidol: A test dose strategy. *Journal of Clinical Psychiatry*, 43(4):157–158, 1982.

Nemiah, J. C.: Dissociative disorders (hysterial neurosis, dissociative type). In H. I. Kaplan, A. M. Freedman, and B. J. Sadock (Eds.), *Comprehensive Textbook of Psychiatry, 3rd Edition*, Volume 2, Baltimore: Williams and Wilkins, 1980.

Nurnberg, H. G., and Suh, R.: Time-limited psychotherapy of the hospitalized borderline patient. *American Journal of Psychotherapy*, 36:82–90, 1982.

Orne, M. T.: The use and misuse of hypnosis in court. *International Journal of Clinical and Experimental Hypnosis*, 27(4):311–341, 1979.

Osborne, M., Crayton, J. W., Javid, J., and Davis, J. M.: Lack of effect of a gluten-free diet on neuroleptic blood levels in schizophrenic patients. *Biological Psychiatry*, 17(5):627–629, 1982.

Peet, M., Bethell, M. S., Coates, A., Khamnee, A. K., Hall, P., Cooper, S. J., King, D. J., and Yates, R. A.: Propranolol in schizophrenia: 1. Comparison of propranolol, chlorpromazine, and placebo. *British Journal of Psychiatry*, 39:105–111, 1981.

Peteet, J. R., and Gutheil, T. G.: The hospital and the borderline patient: Management guidelines for the community mental health center. *Psychiatric Quarterly*, 51(2):106–118, 1979.

Phillips, J. A.: Narcissistic personality. In J. R. Lion (Ed.), *Personality Disorders: Diagnosis and Management*, 2nd Edition. Baltimore: Williams and Wilkins, 1981.

Pickard Vartanian, F., Bunney, W. E., Maier, H. P., Gastpar, M. T., Prakash, R., Sethi, B. B., Lideman, R., Belyaev, B. S., Tsutsulkovaskaja, M. V. A., Jungkunz, G., Netopil, N., Verhoeven, W., and van Praag, H. M.: Short-term naloxone administration in schizophrenic and manic patients: A World Health Organization collaborative study. *Archives of General Psychiatry*, 39:313–318, 1982.

Reid, W. H.: The sadness of the psychopath. *American Journal of Psychotherapy*, 32(4), 1978.

Reid, W. H.: Antisocial personality and related syndromes. In J. R. Lion (Ed.), *Personality Disorders: Diagnosis and Management*. Baltimore: Williams and Wilkins, 1981a.

Reid, W. H. (Ed.): *The Treatment of Antisocial Syndromes*. New York: Van Nostrand Reinhold, 1981b.

Reid, W. H., Ahmed, I., and Levie, C. A.: Treatment of sleepwalking: A controlled study. *American Journal of Psychotherapy*, 35(1):27–37, 1981.

Reid, W. H., and Gutnik, B. D.: Organic treatment of chronically violent patients. *Psychiatric Annals*, 12(5):526–532, 1982.

Reid, W. H., Haffke, E. A., and Chu, C. C.: Diazepam in treatment of intractable sleepwalking. *Hillside Journal of Clinical Psychiatry*, in press.

Reid, W. H., and Matthews, W.: A wilderness experience treatment program for antisocial offenders. *International Journal of Offender Therapy and Comparative Criminology*, 24(2):171–178, 1980.

Reid, W. H., and Solomon, G. H.: Community-based offender programs. In W. H. Reid (Ed.), *The Treatment of Antisocial Syndromes*. New York: Van Nostrand Reinhold, 1981.

Rickels, K., Case, W. G., and Diamond, L.: Relapse after short-term therapy in neurotic outpatients. *International Pharmacopsychiatry*, 15:186–192, 1980.

Robey, A.: Personal communication, 1981.

Ross, W. D., Schultz, J. R., and Edelstein, P.: The biopsychosocial approach: Clinical examples from a consultation-liaison service. *Psychosomatics*, 23(2):141–151, 1982.

Sadivoy, J., Silver, D., and Book, H. E.: Negative responses of the borderline to inpatient treatment. *American Journal of Psychotherapy*, 33(3):404–416, 1979.

Snaith, R. P., and Collins, S. A.: Five exhibitionists and a method of treatment. *British Journal of Psychiatry*, 138:126–130, 1981.

Socarides, C. W.: Some problems encountered in the psychoanalytic treatment of overt male homosexuality. *American Journal of Psychotherapy*, 33(4):506–520, 1979.

Sorensen, T. A.: A follow-up study of operated transsexual females. *Acta Psychiatrica Scandinavica*, 64:50–64, 1981.

Stern, S. L., Rush, A. J., and Mendels, J.: Toward a rational pharmacotherapy of depression. *American Journal of Psychiatry*, 137(5):545–552, 1980.

Stone, W. N., and Gustafson, J. P.: Technique in group psychotherapy of narcissistic and borderline patients. *International Journal of Group Psychotherapy*, 32:29–47, 1982.

Strain, J. J.: Diagnostic considerations in the medical setting. *Psychiatric Clinics of North America*, 4(2):287–300, 1981.

Strider, F. D., and Menolascino, F. J.: Treatment of antisocial syndromes in the mentally retarded. In W. H. Reid (Ed.), *The Treatment of Antisocial Syndromes*. New York: Van Nostrand Reinhold, 1981.

Stürup, G.K., and Reid, W. H.: Herstedvester: An historical overview of institutional treatment. In W. H. Reid (Ed.), *The Treatment of Antisocial Syndromes*. New York: Van Nostrand Reinhold, 1981.

Talbott, J. A.: Chronic mental illness. *Audio Digest Psychiatry*, Volume 11, No. 2, January, 1982.

Tarachow, S.: *An Introduction to Psychotherapy*. New York: International Universities Press, 1963.

Theorell, T.: Life events and manifestations of ischemic heart disease: Epidemiological and psychophysiological aspects. *Psychotherapy and Psychosomatics*, 34:135–148, 1980.

Thigpen, C. H., and Cleckley, H. M.: *The Three Faces of Eve*. New York: McGraw-Hill, 1957.

Tupin, J. P.: Histronic personality. In J. R. Lion (Ed.), *Personality Disorders: Diagnosis and Management*, 2nd Edition. Baltimore: Williams and Wilkins, 1981.

van Kammen, D. P., Docherty, J. T., Marder, S. R., Schulz, S. C., Dalton, L., and Bunney, W. E.: Antipsychotic effects of pimozide in schizophrenia: Treatment response prediction with acute dextroamphetamine response. *Archives of General Psychiatry*, 39:261–266, 1982.

Verhoeven, W. M. A., van Ree, J. M., Heezius-van Bentum, A., de Wied, D., and van Praag, H. M.: Antipsychotic properties of Des-Enkephalin-(Gamma) endorphin in treatment of schizophrenic patients. *Archives of General Psychiatry*, 39:648–654, 1982.

Walsh, V., and Golins, G.: *Exploration of the Outward Bound Process*. Denver: Colorado Outward Bound School, 1976.

Weissman, M. M., Klerman, G. L., Prusoff, B. A., Sholomskas, D., and Padian, N.: Depressed outpatients: Results of one year after treatment with drugs and/or interpersonal psychotherapy. *Archives of General Psychiatry*, 38:51–55, 1981.

Wolpe, J.: Behavior therapy for psychosomatic disorders. *Psychosomatics*, 21(5):379–385, 1980.

Wray, I., and Dickerson, M. G.: Cessation of high frequency gambling and "withdrawal" symptoms. *British Journal of Addiction*, 76:401–405, 1981.

Yesavage, J. A., Becker, J., Werner, P. D., Mills, M. J., Holman, C. A., and Cohn, R.: Serum level monitoring of thiothixene in schizophrenia: Acute single-dose levels at fixed doses. *American Journal of Psychiatry*, 139(2):174–178, 1982.

Name Index

Subject Index